THE PURPLE BUTTERFLY

Susan Hibberd studied at the Dorset Institute of Higher Education before being awarded a BA at Southampton University. After almost a decade as an Internal Auditor in the Civil Service, she gave up full-time work, and now works part-time as a school librarian, which allows her to devote time to her creative interests. She lives in Kent with her daughter and three cats, where she is well-known for her papermaking and community art work.

The Purple Butterfly

Susan Hibberd

The Diggory Press

British Library Cataloguing In Publication Data
A Record of this Publication is available
from the British Library

ISBN 1846851114
978-1-84685-111-7

First published in Great Britain in April 2006
by Diggory Press, an imprint of
Meadow Books, 35 Stonefield Way,
Burgess Hill, West Sussex, RH15 8DW
Website: www.diggorypress.com

Acknowledgements

There are two sets of people to thank in this section - those who have supported me through these strange, unexpected events and those who have helped to make this book possible

Firstly, Colin, my partner, and Claire, my daughter, for their personal support. I know you both had your own stuff to work through as well.

Secondly, to Judith, Grant and Melanie for their encouragement to publish.

Thirdly Katie, who falls into both categories.

Thank you.

Foreword

This is a book about thyroid cancer and its treatment, and it comes in two parts.

The first section, 'The Purple Butterfly', gives an insight into the mind of someone undergoing treatment for a life-threatening disease. I hope it will be read by those who support cancer patients, and lead to a better understanding of the emotional journey they are about to undertake.

The second part 'Flying with the Purple Butterfly', is written for people undergoing radioiodine treatment. This is not given to every thyroid cancer patient, but if you are one of the people who need it, you should read this part of the book.

My advice to you all? Take every bit of help offered, and look to the future.

Sue

The Purple Butterfly

Introduction

I had long-since ceased to notice the lump in my neck, as it had been diagnosed as benign, but my doctor advised me to have it removed anyway. When I started to write this diary, it was only as a way to pass the time while I underwent a routine operation and convalesced for a couple of weeks.

Once I was diagnosed with cancer, I realised the cathartic effect it was having. Seeing things evolve on the screen helped me to organise and process the information I was suddenly presented with, and had previously been mentally blocking. I would urge anyone with cancer to start a diary.

2003 was an odd year for me, and I am still battling with the fall-out. What is has taught me is that we all have a limited amount of time together, and that we need to make the most of that time. I don't feel that my life has been totally transformed, but I do now have a great ability to put things in perspective, and this has made me a much calmer person.

I hope that by reading this, others in the same situation can see that there is light at the end of the tunnel. There doesn't have to be a cure, there just has to be acceptance.

Dramatis personae:

Me	part-time school librarian, part-time papermaker
Colin	my partner, part-time psychiatric nurse, part-time sculptor
Claire	my daughter, part-time teenager, part-time young lady

And some of my friends ..

Judith	fellow thyroid cancer sufferer, who now lives in Holland
Lesley	breast cancer survivor
Helen	long-time thyroid cancer sufferer
Janet	colleague, friend and neighbour
Julie	friend and colleague
Bob & Julia	friends and artists
Kathy	thyroid cancer sufferer from online support group

March - a month of seedlings and birdsong, in which we meet our heroine.

24th March

Dad's birthday. Sent a card. Haven't gone to visit this year, due to being TOO BUSY! Still trying to get house sorted out from the move, and now I have to go into hospital. What bad timing! I just have to breathe calmly, and look through it to the other side, when I will be out, and fit, and able to get on with organising things how I want them. And I will also have a beautiful neck, of course. Goitre-free and swan-like in its perfection.

25th March

All packed and ready to go. My desk at work is all tidied, and I've left notes for the girl who will be looking after my Job for me while I'm away. I hope she doesn't change too many things around. But then again, how much damage can she do in two weeks? It'll be the holiday soon, and there'll be no-one there anyway. I'll sweep in and change it all back again afterwards! Ha!

I've been waiting since October for this operation, and they only sent the letter through three weeks ago with the appointment. You'd think they could get a bit more organised than that, wouldn't you?

I've never been in hospital before. How bad can it be?

26th March

Today I have come into hospital to have my throat cut. I have had this lump in my neck for so many years now that I don't even see it when I look in the mirror. I suppose it's like wearing glasses – sometimes you barely even register the fact. I have to admit that you can see it in photographs, though.

The GP has advised me to have it done 'while I'm still young' (is 44 still young?) so that I can recuperate reasonably quickly, rather than waiting until it gets really large, and I am so much older that my body won't be able to stand the shock of the operation. I don't know what made me agree. I think it's because she's a nice lady and I trust her!

I feel like a bit of a fraud in here. The nurse has shown me to a bed and wandered off. I don't know what I should be doing. There is a leaflet itemising the different types of nurse and their respective uniforms. I'll never remember all those! Do you think it matters if I speak to the wrong one? Everyone else in here is really ill except for me.

The operation is scheduled for 10am tomorrow. I wish it was earlier – all that time to sit and worry about it. The consultant has been round and read me my rights – well, his rights anyway. I have signed to say that he's allowed to do what he wants, and I won't sue. Those aren't the exact words on the paper, but that's what they really mean. He has explained that I might come out with a changed voice, or possibly with no voice at all, but says this is a 'very small' risk. The only thing I am really worried about is whether or not they are going to loose my glasses during the operation, and I am going to wake up and not be able to see anything.

27th March

Throat cut. Tubes everywhere. Colin and Claire came to visit in the evening, and I was too ill to appreciate it. I was quite glad when they went, and I could lie back and wallow in feeling sorry for myself again. Claire brought me a cuddly animal to go in my bed. Surprisingly comforting.

28th March

Loads better today. I think I was still feeling the effects of the anaesthetic yesterday, and I slept all night, even though it was very uncomfortable. I like to sleep on my front or my side, and now I can only sleep on my back. Had porridge for breakfast today. Nice and smooth – no chewing involved.

When the surgeon came yesterday, he told me that he had taken out a large lump on the right side of my thyroid, but that the left side had seemed OK, so he had left it alone. This means that I will still make my own thyroxine, and don't need to take tablets for the rest of my life. I am glad about that. I don't like taking tablets.

The nurse is coming this afternoon to disconnect the two drain tubes that have been left in my chest. They each run down to a vacuum bottle, one either side of my bed, so I am effectively pinned down. It's fun when I want to go to the toilet, as I have to gather them up, and take them with me, as well as the drip-on-a-stick. My neck is all bandaged up, but is not painful.

One of the nurses helped me to have a bath. I got to sit in one of those mechanised chairs that swings over the bath and lowers you in. Made me feel like an old lady. The nurse had to help me wash my back, which had dried blood on it from where one of the drains had leaked (call the plumber!). I can't move my arms about much because it pulls on the stitches, let alone reach behind me to wash.

I was rather hesitant about buzzing for a nurse to help me to the toilet etc a first, but now I am getting used to it. I had a vague feeling that it was only for emergencies (having only ever seen one used on Casualty when the machines in ICU start bleeping), but I realise now that there is very little constant checking on patients, and that they rely on you to ring when you want something. Thank goodness one of the other patients on the ward is a nurse, and I can follow her lead as to what is acceptable.

I was sick this afternoon, but I'm not sure why that was. Could be the anaesthetic, or just the effect of the operation. Perhaps it was the porridge. Limited myself to a sandwich and soup for tea. I dipped the sandwich in the soup to make it soggy, so I didn't need to chew. Comforting by being warm, and also comforting by allowing me to revert to sucking as a means of getting food.

They have told me that they are short of beds, and I have to go somewhere else if I want to stay in hospital. I can hardly move, let alone walk, but I agree. Years of doing as I am told are paying off (for them).

29th March

OK, so I did come home yesterday. They moved me to a private room in The Rotary Suite. Very nice room, separate bathroom, but so lonely! I was there all afternoon, and only saw a nurse once. When you are on the normal ward there are nurses everywhere, and you know that you are being looked after. I hated it, so Colin came and brought me home. What a lot of paperwork to do! I suppose they have to cover themselves in the event of any complaint, but still.....! They have given me some dressings for the District Nurse to change when she comes and visits.

So this is what it's like to feel old. I am suffering from lack of sleep, but I am also very stiff. That's the worst thing about this. I don't know if it's what they did to me, or the stress of it all, or because I am holding myself rigid to protect the stitches. I have to be helped in and out of the bath. Still feeling a bit ill, but I think that is because of the tiredness – I never was very good at going without sleep. I don't want to get old and infirm. I don't want to be blind, or lose the use of my legs, but most of all, I don't want to be incapable of looking after myself.

They have given me Paracetamol for the pain, but there really isn't much. I read that this is because they have cut through all the nerves. Mostly, I just feel sick. I feel quite brave about coping so well.

30th March

Mother's Day, and for the first time in years, I haven't sent a card. If I'd have thought about it, I'd have sent one before I went it. Never mind. Claire brings me a CD.

I have found that as well as not being able to tip my head back, I can't bend it forward either. This means that I can't bend to pick things up, or get into and out of the bath. You don't realise the ways your body works until it stops doing it. When I want to get out of the bath, I turn onto my front, and get up via all fours. This avoids any strain on my poor neck. Never let it be said that I can be beaten!

I have perfected the technique of getting a drink by putting my hand under the tap like a caveman or a monkey. Before the operation, I'd likely as not stick my head under the tap to rinse my mouth out when cleaning my teeth. Now I can't bend forward like that, I have to scoop the water up. When I first did it, it all ran through my fingers, but now I am a dab hand at it.

31st March

Flowers arrive from work. That's nice, even if the money is only given because it's easier than saying 'no' to a keen colleague with an envelope. Is that cynical of me?

My parents came today to visit me. I did find that it was a strain to be nice, like it was when I got visitors in hospital. Even though I am the ill person, and they are here to help, I feel that I have to be polite and jolly. At least my house has had a good clean, though! Not only that, but my Dad has cut the grass for me! Hooray! Mother washed my hair while I leaned over the bath. That brought back memories. It was nice to just give myself up to someone else's ministrations. I stood where I was told, and moved when I was told. Nicely insular and catatonic.

They brought a camp bed with them, and I am sleeping on that now. It won't fit in my bedroom, so it is set up in the front room. The reason I like it, is because the back can be raised, so that I can sleep sitting up. This is much more com fortable that lying flat on my back. I can't move my head from side to side, and it makes the back of my head hurt. I feel like a Victorian lady with consumption, lying on my bed in the living room, with visitors trailing past. Not as romantic as Emily Bronte, lying on her cold couch in a chilly Yorkshire rectory, of course. I think, given the choice, I'd prefer a longer-term and less fatal illness. Just enough to keep me from doing anything too strenuous, but not enough to inconvenience me if I felt like doing anything. Something where I had good days and bad days would be fine. Something much easier to bear than what I have now, anyway.

Feeling very poorly and sorry for myself.

April – the month of fools - the plot begins to thicken

1st April

The District Nurse came today, and brought a trainee with her who was a girl I had known when she was younger. That was very odd. Suddenly, instead of me being the grown-up, and she the child, we reversed roles. I was the taking advice from her instead of vice versa. I suppose that will happen to me more and more often as people I knew as children grow up. Something to think about later.

I had some of the steri-strips taken off my neck. It was an odd sensation, and made me feel a bit sick. It didn't hurt, but I had the irrational fear that the stitches would be pulled open and start to bleed. I haven't got over the thought of the little cartoon man on the toothpaste advert with the flip-top head. That could so easily be me. I'm sure that's how they did the operation. Anyway, she has re-applied the dressing, and is coming back in a few days time to take the remaining strips off. I still haven't seen what it looks like. It seemed odd to hear them talk about it as a 'wound'. I always think of a wound as being a mistake, and a bit of an emergency, not a planned cut. There is a bit of thread still loose, but she thinks it is a dissolvable stitch, and that it will disappear on its own.

It's really odd being at home, knowing that everyone else is at work. I worked out how to unclip the shower screen today, so that I can run a bath for myself. It's one of those things you don't ever learn to do if you can do without it.

Colin had to come in when I had finished and support me while I stepped out. I am so frightened of falling, or of wrenching my neck somehow. I know it's wimpy, but I'm still going to do it. The nurse didn't put the padded bandage back on, and I have looked at it I the mirror. I look awful! My face is all grey and puffy. The cut itself is not too bad, if a little pink.

2nd April

I have been left all alone today. I woke up to make sure Claire went to school on time, and then slept a bit more. It takes so long to do things – it reminds me so much of Julie's stories of her elderly grandmother taking twenty-five minutes to dress. It takes me about that long now.

But the good news is that I am losing weight! I am now down to 9st 2lb, which is the lightest I have been for about four years. Let's hope I can keep it off now I've finally got rid of it.

3rd April

The nurse called again today (sans assistant), and took off the remaining strips across the wound (as I now know to call it). She said it looked rather red, and advised me to call the doctor out to look. The doctor phoned and asked me to go into the surgery, rather than him coming out to me. Like a fool, I agreed, and paid for a taxi to go down there. He has given me 7 days worth of antibiotics. I put the bandage on again to go to the surgery, in case I frightened the other patients by going in there looking like Mrs Frankenstein.

I wish I had a pound for everyone who'd told me to keep my chin up, and then giggled. I don't think I've heard the same joke repeated so much in a long time.

4th April

This morning there was a power cut. It was very odd to lie in bed and her nothing. Just the twittering of gathering swallows in the skies – oh, no, that's autumn. Just the tweeting of birds in the trees, and the occasional shout of a child playing. Very rural. Very pre-war. Idyllic? Only on the telly. The power came on again in a hour or so, and the pneumatic drills, appliances, and radios started again. Life back to normal. Better go and reset all the clocks.

This afternoon, I walked across to the shop opposite my house, and down to the post-box at the end of my road – all of 20 yards away. I put the bandage around my neck to go, and walked very slowly, so as not to joggle my neck. I was surprised to find how worried I was that I might fall over. I don't know if it's the thought that it would cause me pain, or the thought that it might all rip open that is the worst. I felt as if everyone was watching me, for some reason. Never mind – at least I was out in the fresh air, even if it was only for three minutes.

5th April

Janet rang today and asked if I needed any shopping done. Luckily, I stocked up on tins and filled the freeze before I went into hospital. The milk gets delivered, and the shop across the road is OK for bread etc. I declined politely, but what I really wanted to ask was whether she'd vacuum upstairs, clean the toilet and take the bins out in the morning. I suppose it's a measure of friendship, how much you ask of people. If I was ever really ill, I suppose I'd have to swallow my pride and just ask.

6th April

I have been sleeping propped up in my own bed now, almost upright. It takes ages arranging the pillows, and they slip down during the night. Someone should invent pillows with Velcro strips down them, so you could make yourself a little cocoon to lie in. I like it best when Colin's on night duty, and I can wake up as many times as I like and throw pillows around without fear of waking him. I really can sympathise with crotchety old ladies who growl at everyone when they are in pain. This is good practice for when I am older.

7th April

Today, I found one of those black-outface masks given to passengers on long-haul flights. I tried it during my afternoon nap, and it has made a surprisingly big difference. I have never been able to sleep with the light on, not even the hall light, so finding this has been a real blessing. I'm like a cat, now, and can doze off at the drop of a hat. In fact, when I sleep during the day, I am usually accompanied by at least one cat; normally more. They are comforting as well as warm.

8th April

Contrary to popular opinion on my housekeeping skills, I have been doing a little light dusting today. What I really want to do is to re-organise my garage. Having only moved house a few weeks before I went into hospital, it's still really muddled in there. I want to make it into a workshop, so I suppose I can plan where I want everything to be, even if I can't physically move anything. Another thing on the list for later.

9th April

The consultant's secretary rang today to change my appointment to the 16th. He must be going on holiday, or have someone more important to see. Never mind, it was nice of her to ring, rather than writing, which is slower and less personal.

10th April

Hooray! Had two lots of visitors today, and they brought chocolates, flowers and cards. It was very odd to speak to lots of people at once, because each time I wanted to look at whoever was speaking, I had to move my whole body, not instead of turning my neck. Another new skill!

11th April

Had to set up an art exhibition today. It was my first real 'outing', and I was a bit wary about going in the car. Rather pathetic, really. Anyway, it was fine, except that I felt bad that I couldn't help much. I couldn't help with heavy things, so I sat and watched for a lot of the time. It was tiring being out of the house all afternoon. 'They' say it's the fresh air, and I am sure 'they' are right.

12th April

Last day at work for everyone else but me. Sad not to be there, but happy that everyone else is on holiday too, now, and I am no different from them.

13th April

Claire's birthday today. Didn't have all the presents etc that I usually do, because I haven't been able to get out. I did get a lot of stuff before I went into hospital (how brilliantly well organised, I hear you cry). She just wanted to be with her friends anyway.

14th April

Preview evening for the art show. Not as many people came as we thought, due to it being in a really out-of-the-way place, but that was good from my point of view. Lots of people asking how I was, which was nice. Colin bought me a lovely long silk scarf, that I threw casually and artistically round my neck to hide the scar. They might have thought I moved rather oddly, but at least they weren't alienated by a big an angry-looking red gash. A perfect solution.

15th April

Drove all the way to Dover today. On my own. Not terribly safe, due to the fact that I can't turn round very easily.

However, I think that the only way to get used to it is to do it more. I shall have to do lots of little safe journeys in the middle of the night to practise. Or perhaps I can practise by sitting in the driveway and doing turning round exercises? That would save on petrol!

16th April

Went to see the doctor this morning to get an extension on my sick note. The present one runs out on a Wednesday, and I want it to go to the Monday afterwards. He was very nice about it, and didn't see a problem.

Appointment with my consultant who in formed me that some 'abnormal cells' had been detected, and that he needed to remove the second half of my thyroid, to be on the safe side. Oh well, more time off work. His secretary is going to write with an appointment, but he said it should be soon.

17th April

Rang Julie at work to let her know I'd be off. Bit difficult when I haven't got a date, but it seems silly to go back in between. Got all the gossip.

18th April

Good Friday. Not so good for me, as I'm still playing catch-up to get my house tidy, and get organised for Easter.

19th April

Went round town today without covering my scar. Felt very brave, and as if everyone was looking at me. I have decided not to cover it up, though, because if I start, I won't know when to stop. I might as well get it out in the open and keep it there.

20th April

Easter Day. Claire isn't here, and I have a day to myself. Now that it isn't that unusual, it isn't really a treat. Time to catch up on the housework.

21st April

The cats have been really nice to me recently. It probably stems from the fact that I feed them on time more often, now. When I sit reading or watching television, they come and sit with me. My favourite one follows me round the house. When I have a bath, she even comes and sits in the washbasin to waits for me. What a sweetie.

22nd April

Tried moving some furniture on my own today. Not a good idea. It was only small stuff (some bedside cabinets), but I can really feel where it has pulled the cut in my neck. When you are convalescing, it is ever so difficult to decide how much resting to do, and how much exercise you should do. There's no alternative but to work until you feel the strain, I suppose.

23rd April

I have ordered a lot of books from the Internet. Since I am stuck here for a while more with nothing to do, I thought I'd treat myself. I have bought lots of 'whodunnit' books, as they are easy to read. When I was really ill, I read nothing, but just watched TV. When I was recovering, I read Ian Rankin and Francis Fyfield. Now I am almost fully better, I can cope with Dennis Lehane and Michael Connolly. I did pick '*Sophie's World*' off the shelf at the library, but I put it back again to save for later, when I can give it my full attention.

24th April

I seem to be much better today. Almost back to my old bouncy self! I suppose I ought to be looking after myself really well now, and getting as fit as I can before the next operation.

Once again, I feel like I am having time off work for no good reason. I should have been going back to work on Monday, but it seems pointless to go back for such a short time. I popped in this afternoon to see how things were, and poked around my desk. I was pleased to see that some of the work hadn't been done as I would have done it. It was nice to talk to people, but not so nice to have to keep repeating things over and over, as different people came up and asked me how I was. Everyone was lovely, though, and says they will be glad when I am back. Not as glad as I'll be!

25th April

I had quite a good day today. I have decided not to worry about being off work. I hardly ever have a day off, and now I'm making up for it. The doctor has signed me off, so it's not like I am pulling a fast one. I got out a tin of paint and did some decorating in my bedroom. It was OK when I did small patches, but I still don't have the full range of movement in my arms. funny how my arms seem to be affected, when it was my neck that was cut. What I mean is, when I move my arms too much, it pulls on my neck. Poor me! By dint of going up and down on a chair and moving it along more than I normally would do, I managed to paint almost a whole wall. When Colin comes home, I will ask him to fill in the high bits.

26th April

Got my overnight case down from the loft and did my packing today. funnily enough, I put in almost the same things as before, so that's one point to me for getting it right first time. The only thing I put in different was an easier book to read.

27th April

Took down the exhibition today. Once again, it made me realise that I am not fully recovered yet. for everyday activities, I am OK, but for cleaning out the garage, and lifting sculptures, I am sorely lacking.

28th April

I should have gone back to work today. I get a few more days holiday than everyone else, so I suppose that makes up for the time I was in bed over Easter.

29th April

Got my bedroom sorted today, with cushions and pillows easily to hand. Moved some things around in the kitchen cupboards so I could get to them without reaching, and put the most frequently used things out on the work surface. All ready now.

30th April

Hmm. Today I had to travel the 45 minutes out to the hospital, and sit almost all afternoon while they did the pre-admission checks, only to be told that they didn't have a bed for me. This means that I am going to have to get up at 6.30am tomorrow to get here in time for the operation. Not a happy bunny. I suppose at least I am going to get it done, and they haven't cancelled altogether.

Once again, the consultant went through the possible risks with me, and explained the operation, and got me to sign on the dotted line. He reminded me about the risk to my voice. It's lucky I understand the rules of probability, and know that there is no more risk to me this time than there was last time. I'm not worried – it didn't happen last time, and I don't expect it will this time either.

May – a month of ribbons and flowers. Final realisation leads our heroine into the Slough of Despond.

1st May

Up at 6.30am to get to hospital on time. At least I know the drill here, as I have come to the same hospital. I know roughly what is going to happen, and in what order. I even know how to put on the tight elasticised socks they make you wear, that stop thrombosis. The trick is to keep the plastic bag they come in, and put that over your foot first, so that the sock will slide up easily.

They sent me up at 8am. They have only put one drain in this time. Was sick as soon as I woke up. Much less intensive nursing this time. I wonder if they are short staffed, or whether they think I know what I am doing this time?

2nd May

Something has been niggling me about yesterday. When I woke up, I was very hot, and realised I had a plastic blanket on me, and there was a space blanket rolled up at the end of my bed. When Colin came to visit, he said he'd been told that there was trouble when I came out of the anaesthetic. When he said that, I remembered briefly regaining consciousness, and then beginning to shake uncontrollably. The plastic blanket that had been left on my bed was an inflatable air bag, and I can remember that they had a large hot air blower that they inflated it with to keep me warm. I suppose I went into shock. Anyway, I am here now, and no-one has mentioned it, so I either it wasn't a big thing, or they are keeping quiet about it. Either way, I don't really care, as long as I made it.

The instructions above my bed have not been changed from the pre-operation instruction of 'sips only', so I have to argue with the tea-lady each time she comes round, to get a cup of tea.

The other ladies in this ward have been chatting to each other, and although I haven't really felt like Joining in, I have been listening. I have decided that the old joke about hospitals being dangerous places to go, because you die there, is actually not that far from the truth. Each lady recounted at least one example of someone who'd come in to hospital for a particular operation, and gone home knowing they had cancer. The patient in the opposite bed to me was one of these people herself. She was clearly very shocked, and kept crying during her whispered conversations with visitors. She then got whisked off into isolation because she'd contracted some contagious disease as well. They came and steam-cleaned her bed, furniture, curtains etc. There but for the grace of God...

The consultant saw me briefly and said he would make an appointment for about 2 weeks time, and that I could go home. This was at about 12 noon. Three extra blood tests were taken mid-afternoon (at three separate times), and by 4pm the Ward Sister had the results, and was waiting for a doctor to confirm whether or not they indicated that medication was necessary. I didn't leave until 6pm. Straight to bed when I got home.

3rd May

The District Nurse called to change the dressing. As it had been changed the day before, on discharge, this was a wasted journey. She made a note on her form that she had been, and left. Never mind, I feel so glad to be at home, in familiar surroundings, (where I control the light switch, and live plants are allowed) that I can cope with anything.

4th May

I notice that I haven't received any flowers from work this time. I suppose the kitty only runs to one bunch per illness.

Not sleeping properly. I've got five pillows and a cushion piled up on my bed to try and keep me upright while I sleep, and they keep slipping down in the night. I have to sleep in the middle of the bed to allow for 'slippage'.

5th May

Visit from the District Nurse (again), who noticed that the wound was red and rather puffy. Does this sound familiar? She phoned the on-call doctor and asked him to visit. He prescribed me 5 days worth of antibiotics. No wonder I am feeling so sick still.

On a very still and clear day, I can hear the trains go past. I don't know why, but that is a sound I love. Perhaps it is a memory from my childhood. Perhaps it is because I like to think of the excitement associated with a train Journey. Anyway, it makes me smile.

6th May

I wonder when I will ever be well again. I am trying to think back to last operation to see how soon I got over it, but I think I have blocked it out, and this diary isn't very detailed. Perhaps I should have written down every single thing.

My neck is now swollen to almost twice its normal size, and my face is an unbecoming shade of grey. The dark purplish lines under my eyes don't help matters at all.

I stay in bed almost all morning, and dress slowly about 10.00 or 11.00. After a few hours up, watching TV, I have to go back to bed. Sometimes I sleep on the sofa. I watch Quincy from 1.30 until 2.30, and have my nap afterwards. I am so lucky that my neck doesn't hurt from the operation although I t aches from where I am holding it in one position all the time.

7th May

Last night I had to call Colin at 3am. I woke up and felt wetness on my chest. It was pus seeping out from under the dressing round my neck. I panicked, and rang him to come and see what he thought. He re-dressed it for me, and I had a drink of hot milk and went back to sleep. This morning we rang the GP, and were told that house calls are in the afternoons only. Colin drove me to the local A&E department, where the nurse 'expressed' the wound. Lucky for me the area is still really numb. I went a bit woozy from the thought of it, as I could still feel her pushing and pressing around it. I had thoughts of it all popping open, and blood gushing out everywhere. She cleaned it as best she could, took a swab, and dressed it again.

The on-call doctor came in the afternoon. He asked me what I had been told about the operation, and I was left feeling that he knew more than he had said, so when he went to wash his hands, I slid the copy of his visiting notes under a magazine. A snooper never hears good of themselves. It told me I have cancer.

8th May

Well, yesterday I found out I have cancer. Papillary thyroid cancer to be exact. I have had two major operations in the last six weeks, my neck is swollen to twice its normal size, and the wound is leaking pus. I am having to take sea-sickness tablets to ease the nausea. Not quite a situation where death would be preferable, but I can see the temptation to think like that. Luckily, in my present sate, I am unable to process the information.

I try to force down the plateful of dinner Colin places in front of me. I feel so guilty that I can't eat it all. I want to make him feel better about the situation, and although I know this isn't the way, it somehow seems important to try. I feel responsible for his state of mind. Should I honour the relationship by trusting him with my fears, or show selfless moral strength by keeping it all to myself?

How do you decide how much to share, and how much to deal with on your own? Unable to decide, I veer between the two.

9th May

Another sleepless night. My shoulders ache from keeping my head in one place, and my back aches from sleeping sitting-up to allow the wound to drain. When I want to sit upright, I grab a handful of hair and pull my head up, so I don't use my neck muscles.

I am very tired all the time, and unable to do some of the most basic of tasks. I step into my tops and pull them up when I dress, because I can't raise my hands over my head. I have difficulty bending over, it's not as bad as when I first came home from hospital, but still worried that I might injure myself further. I climb carefully into the bath in the evenings, and think that this must be what it is like to be old. I dread the day when I can't do things for myself. At the moment, I am ill for a short period of time, and people are glad to help. Would they be so glad to help if it was a permanent disability? I feel like I am gradually getting slower and slower at things. Soon, it should improve, and I will be on the mend. I hope.

10th May

How do you tell people you have cancer? What do you tell them? Who do you tell? I realize I am woefully unaware of any of the facts about my condition. I want some hard and fast rules and statistics to pass on – there are none.

I spend hours searching the Internet for answers, and all I do is come up with more and more questions. One question I DON'T ask is 'why me?' A lot of words are devoted to causes and explanations – I skip past these pieces – all I want to know is 'Will I die?'. I cannot find an answer.

11th May

I rang my mother today and told her the news. I felt guilty and selfish, having been brought up on a diet of Girls Own stories of selfless stiff-upper-lip heroism. I tried to think what it would be like if Claire had told me she had cancer, and couldn't do it. In the end, I compromised. I allowed myself the luxury of complaining my mummy that I didn't feel well, at the expense of her peace of mind. I comforted myself with the thoughts that you can't protect everyone else all of the time – you have to see to your own needs, and that she would have found out soon enough anyway.

Colin has been telling his family about my illness – I think it helps him to share. The word 'cancer' is such a monster in the cupboard that it helps to have it in the open. Also, if you don't tell people straight away, when do you tell them? There is never a 'good' time. A 'Get Well Soon' card arrives from his daughters. A nice thought, but somehow it doesn't quite cover it....

12th May

A trip to the doctors for more antibiotics. She talks about the cancer, and watches for my reaction. I am surprised that I feel tearful talking about it. I suppose I should find time to think it through, and stop burying it. I smile, and shrug off her concern. Of course I am OK, I'm an intelligent woman. Doesn't that make me more able to cope than most people? She prescribed another 7 days of antibiotics for the continuing wound infection.

I cry a lot now.

13th May

Today I have joined an Internet support group. I read an entry on the message board saying 'If anyone talks about the Internet being useless, ask them if they have ever had cancer'. I have found having access to a world of information invaluable, especially the first-hand experience of other people with thyroid cancer. I get stuck in, asking the most basic of questions, and am soon getting to grips with the medical jargon. This means I can interpret articles in online medical journals, as well as on people's home pages.

14th May

There is a tree of white lilac flowers outside my bedroom window. I have pulled the net curtain back, and am lying on my bed, watching it move in the wind. The huge, heavy blossoms bob and nod, spectacular in size, elegant in colour, their intricate texture and sensual shape making an irresistible show. I think that perhaps I could ask for lilacs at my funeral, and imagine them piled untidily over a glossy hardwood coffin. Lady of the Camellias, eat your heart out.

15th May

Finally, I have told Claire about the cancer. After a few brief questions, she carried on watching the television. Was she devastated and hiding it well, or did she just not care? I think perhaps I made too light of it, in an effort not to scare her too much. I think it is OK that I did that. Time enough to worry her later, if I get really ill.

16th May

I have found out that about 1,100 people a year are diagnosed with thyroid cancer in the UK, and that a lot more have it but never know about it. This is because it is so slow-growing that they die of something else first, and it is only discovered if an autopsy is performed. 250 people die of it every year. If only there was a way of telling if you were going to be one of these.

Colin is beginning to get annoyed with me talking about thyroid cancer all the time. He thinks it would be healthier for me to forget it for a while, and to concentrate on something else. I can't. It is all I think about from when I get up, until the time I go to bed. When I am doing something else, I keep my mind on that, but whenever my mind wanders, when I am watching tv, dusting, or walking to the shop, it keeps going over and over the in formation that I have. I am not well enough yet to do too much, so I tend to spend a lot of time on the computer, looking up more and more facts. People do say that information gives you power.

17th May

In the two weeks preceding treatment by radioactive iodine, many doctors advise that you follow an iodine-free diet. The idea is that starving the remaining thyroid tissue of iodine will make it more likely to suck up the radioactive iodine when it does get some. Like offering a sugar-coated pill. Death in a pretty package. The tissue is then poisoned, and gradually dies off. Doctors can then more easily target remaining areas of malignant tissue. I am glad there is some positive action I can take, rather than sitting around, waiting.

18th May

I have been looking around the shops for ready-prepared food to eat on my low iodine diet (LID), because I don't think I will feel like cooking while I am ill. Gosh, it's hard! Why do they put salt in cakes? We do seem to be better off than the Americans, though, and I even found a chocolate-covered rice cake that is OK in the diet – yum!

I wrote to the major supermarket chains to ask if they could help me find iodine-free foods. I feel as if I have achieved something now I have started my list of LID food. When it is finished, I can offer copies to other people.

My friend wrote:

> *You've been fantastic - having the energy and the inclination - at the same time trying to deal with the scary diagnosis of thyroid cancer.*
> *Kathy*

This pleased me. I am glad that someone thinks I am 'fantastic'. It certainly doesn't feel like that from the inside. I also think that doing to booklet is a way of avoiding having to think about having cancer. If I can keep myself busy until they've got rid of it all, I think I will have got through this well. Of course, I will always have the knowledge that it could come back at any time, but at least it won't be inside me, and such a threat to my life that they have to do the treatment almost immediately.

19th May

I have written to my GP to get a copy of my notes, and an exemption certificate. Now I am on Thyroxine for the rest of my life, I don't have to pay prescription charges. It's funny to think that I would die if I stopped taking the Thyroxine. I can understand quite easily about dying from cancer, as bits of me stop working. I wonder how long it would take to die of lack of Thyroxine? What would the symptoms be?

Every now and then, I get a fit of crying. I think perhaps I should start to drink more to make up for all the lost fluid. I don't know if this means that I am bottling it up. I don't feel like I am. Perhaps it would be healthier to cry a little bit every day, rather than buckets and buckets every couple of weeks. Perhaps it would be healthier not to have cancer in the first place.

20th May

I am amazed at how much energy I have. Even though I am still tired at the end of each day, I feel better than I ever did before. Thyroid cancer is very slow-growing, and I think I have had it for years – maybe even decades? I look at photographs of me before I had the operations, and see the size of the swelling in my neck. It amazes me that I never thought of the possibility of it being malignant before. There is a very fine line to tread between having a reasonable amount of confidence in the professional competence of the medical profession, and such a blind faith in their superiority that it blocks all common sense.

21st May

This afternoon I had an appointment to see the surgeon, so that he could explain what he has done. He does not realise I already know I have cancer.

He told me I have/had thyroid carcinoma. Even he can't use the 'C' word. He says that he has cut it all out, and is referring me on to another hospital for radiation treatment. I tried to ask about survival rates, but felt awkward being so direct, and allowed myself to be put off by vague speculation on his part.

I came out dazed. He is not the first doctor to tell me that I have cancer, and yet I am still shocked. I feel empty-headed, and wonder if I heard correctly.

22nd May

I have re-read my copy of the Guideline for the Management of Thyroid Cancer in Adults today, published by the British Thyroid Association and the Royal College of Physicians. I was looking especially at the procedures for radioiodine (RAI) treatment. Injected with radioactive iodine, and put in a lead-lined room until the Geiger counter shows I am safe, apparently. Still better than chemotherapy, though. How lucky I am to have this type of cancer. How unlucky to have cancer at all.

I read that in the US, one session of RAI costs $8,000. Hurrah for the NHS.

23rd May

I am still finding it hard to come to terms with having cancer. How many weeks has it been now? I have written to my consultant asking for him to write to me so I can see it in black-and-white, and I can hold it and read it. Part of me is still in denial, and I feel someone is going to come along and say 'WHAT?! Go back to work, and stop being so stupid!'

24th May

I have noticed a surprising number of Internet sites offering 'cures' for various types of cancer. I can understand that diet, exercise or relaxation can help boost the bodies own immune system, and help it fight back, but companies offering pills that cure are downright liars. They should not be allowed to make money from other people's fears. I am tempted to investigate some of the alternative therapies offering relief. It merely goes to show that although I don't normally use any of their systems or products, I am suddenly as sad and desperate as the next person. When it comes to it, we are all the same. However high our moral stance from the safety of an ordinary world, we would all fight for the last crumbs or the last place in the lifeboat when it came to it.

I have emailed a lot of people to let them know that I am ill. I don't know what prompted me to do it, but I have found it very useful in helping me to come to terms with it. It makes it more real. I'm still not brave enough to ring people up and tell them, although I am getting quite good at telling people I meet face-to-face. Having had two operations helps, because I can bring the fact that I have cancer into the conversation as an explanation for that, rather than as a topic in its own right. This sort of gets it said, without making it a major issue. I do feel that I owe it to people to tell them. I would be offended if one of my friends had cancer and didn't tell me.

Somehow, the people from my past seem very important to me now. Perhaps it is the need to reaffirm what I know, to set it against the uncertainty of my future. I feel like a person in a suddenly darkened room, feeling around for something solid that I recognise. I need to get my bearings again, before I can continue to live my life. I have made contact with people I have not spoken to for years, as if I was checking for parts of my house after an earthquake. And it's OK – life is still as it was before the bombshell. It's me that is different, once I can acknowledge and accept that, I can move on.

25th May

I am very grateful for the support of the other people on the Internet message board. As I learn more, and am even able to answer other people's questions. It makes me feel more in control of something that is, at this stage, still unknown. I could be dead in ten years time.

26th May

Lunch with three girls from work. Two of them know I have cancer, but I don't know if the other one has been told. I tried to slip it into the conversation, and failed miserably. The longer I leave it, the harder it is to backtrack. Eventually, I gave up, and the conversation moved on. I hope she doesn't think I didn't want to trust her with the in formation, and take offence. There is a delicate line between wanting people to know, and a fear of pushing yourself forward. How do you judge if someone will be pleased that you shared with them, or annoyed that you are making a fuss? I suppose, in the end, it doesn't really matter.

27th May

I have been cutting the front garden hedge in stages, tackling a three-foot run at a time. I can only manage 10-15 minutes, and then I need a rest. I keep the shears by the front door – I hope I get it finished before the first bit needs doing again!

I'm beginning to get a bit angry now that this cancer wasn't spotted earlier. Am I justified in feeling like this? How can you tell whether anyone was negligent or not? What difference would it make if they were? I can't go back and change anything. It's not like taking your car back to be mended a second time. Now I have got this, I am stuck with it. forever.

28th May

I met a friend's children at the shops today, and they asked about my scar. I told them I had had an operation, and left it at that. I felt like I was lying to them by telling them a half-truth. Are you protecting children when you keep things from them, or setting them up for a harder fall later on, when life's realities become apparent to them? Who knows?

29th May

My sister visited today, and brought me some relaxation tapes. I know they will improve my life by relaxing me, and I think about whether they could perform a deeper function. Worth investigating? Probably.

30th May

What's a good age to die? If the doctor diagnoses me at Stage III, then I have only a 70% chance of living another ten years. This means I have could die in my mid-fifties. Is that an acceptable life-span? Probably not. If I live another twenty years, and die in my mid-sixties, is that an acceptable life-span? After all, it's almost three-score-years-and-ten. I think I should expect to live to about 75-80. I wouldn't like to be ill for too long before I die.

Aren't statistics funny? I wonder what the chances are of dying from being run over by a bus in the next ten years? It makes a big difference if you say the figures round the other way. 70% chance of survival sounds quite good – getting on for 100%, I'd say. 30% chance of dying sounds bad – it's almost a third. That's one in three. It all hangs on whether the cancer has taken over other parts of my body. You can do without your thyroid – they just cut it out and replace the hormones it produces with chemicals. Some things can't be cut out.

The thing is, whatever stage the doctor allocates to my particular situation, I am still left wondering. There are no absolutes. I will know if I am in a high, medium or low risk category, and exactly what level of risk that is, but I shan't know if I am going to die or not. I will never know that. Perhaps I should stop worrying and get on with it. I'd be annoyed if I suddenly became terminally ill without having done the stuff I wanted to.

June – the month of honeybees and blossom, in which we talk of blood, sweat and tears.

1st June

I bought a bread-maker today, so I don't have to eat commercially-produced bread in the run-up to my RAI. Apparently, they use iodine in the processing of the flour, as well as in the dough conditioners. I've been wanting a bread-maker for a long time, and felt unable to justify the expense. Thank goodness I now have thyroid cancer and can have one!

2nd June

Spoke today to the secretary at the Nuclear Medicine Department at the hospital I will be attending. It is SO GOOD to hear someone talking with authority about thyroid cancer. My spirits have lifted, and I can feel myself smiling again. At last I have found someone who knows how to help me. Someone is going to take my hand and lead me out of this. The psychological boost it gives me is indescribable. Appointment booked for Monday June 9th!

3rd June

Someone in the Internet support group asks about a colour for thyroid cancer, as breast cancer has taken pink. Someone else suggests purple, the colour of iodine.

4th June

Another brief chat with the surgeon. I came out feeling dissatisfied, again, and I have cancelled my sixth-months appointment with him. I have told him my fears, and he seems unable to sympathize or acknowledge them, let alone alleviate them. He tells me that it is impossible to offer a prognosis at this stage. I realize that must be the case, before any scans etc have been done, but surely my asking about it must mean that I am worried. I wanted him to discuss the best and worst case scenarios, and let me know the probabilities at least. Oh well…

5th June

I found out today that having Hashimoto's Thyroiditus (which means I produce antibodies against the thyroid functions) means that the annual test they do to check whether they cancer has returned can be unreliable. Great. So I carry on, and wait for a lump to show, do I? It goes on my list of questions for the doctor.

Got a letter from the vague surgeon, confirming his diagnosis of thyroid carcinoma, and saying that 'At the moment, it is confined to the thyroid'. Well, that's fine, because my thyroid is in a glass jar in a laboratory somewhere! It won't be annoying me any more! Or will it?

6th June

All-time low today. I started looking up details of funeral arrangements on the Internet. A standard funeral costs £1,800, and can be booked in advance. I was tempted, but have decided to save up. I stopped short of choosing hymns.

I was meant to go to a party this evening, but I couldn't face it. I have had enough of people asking how I am, and feeling that I have to reply 'I'm fine' in my best airhostess voice. I know it is the only option when you don't know someone very well, but I do feel like telling them outright – ' I have cancer, I feel awful, I don't know yet if I'm going to die, and I have months to go before the doctors can tell me - OK?' I decided to stay away altogether rather than make a fool of myself by being rude to someone.

7th June

I have been watching City Hospital on television. Although I realise that I am seriously ill, and that I don't yet know exactly how ill I am, or have a definite prognosis, I can still be glad that I don't have something yucky, painful or disfiguring. Even the treatment isn't particularly bad. This is why some people call it 'the good cancer'.

8th June

My weight has dropped 10lb since the last operation on 1st May. This is the lightest I have been for years. If I had the energy to tone it up instead of looking like a cross between a scrunchie and a rag doll, I'd be laughing. As it is, I can still only exercise in short bursts.

Started passing out copies of my LID list to other English people. I am so glad to be able to help. I have been off work for so long now, I am beginning to feel really useless. Tomorrow I will find out if it is worth going back.

9th June

Received a copy of the histology report for my second operation through the post this morning. The piece they took out measured 7cm x 5 cm x 2 cm. Add this to the piece they took out last time, and you have a cancerous lump about the size of an audiocassette box. In addition to this they also removed a benign tumour about the size of a ping-pong ball. No wonder I've lost weight!!

Visit to the Nuclear Medicine Department, and a chat with the consultant. My faith in human nature has been restored. I am happy to have this man treat me, and am confident that he is able to make a difference. He has explained what I have, and how they propose to treat it. We talked about the fact that he can't offer a prognosis at this stage, but he has explained why, and when it will be possible. This is so much better than my vague surgeon. I don't expect the doctors to have all the answers at once, but I do expect them to know how to go about getting them.

Came home and started immediately on the LID. At last, something I have control over. I feel capable and somehow morally superior as I tuck into chicken salad (with dressing, not mayonnaise!), and fresh fruit salad.

10th June

Went into work today, and felt bad that I was in such a good mood. Good job I've got a huge unhealed scar across my neck, or they wouldn't have believed I was ill at all. I am so glad it's all getting sorted out, that I am running on adrenaline. I also think my body is now functioning as it should do, after years of fighting the cancer growing inside it. No wonder I've always been so tired and lacking in energy.

Colin has bought me a little figure of a rabbit called Hope. I keep her by my bedside, and look at her. She is reaching her arms up, and has a big smile on her face. I'll be like that again one day.

11th June

Had a bone scan today. They injected radioactive technetium into me at 9.30am and told me to go away and drink eight glasses of water before I came back for the scan at 12.30pm. Have you any idea how difficult that is? I understand it is necessary to push the stuff round my body, but it's not easy! By 11.30am I was feeling sick, and slowed down. It was worth it, though. Twenty minutes laying on a hard narrow ironing board, while a machine the size of a small dishwasher hovers 2cm above your nose is not fun.

When it had passed my neck, I was told I could move my head, and watched the skeleton (MY skeleton) appearing on the screen. It looked OK to me, but a second screen showed lines and lines of multicoloured data, which I could not read, and wouldn't have been able to interpret anyway. Afterwards, I was told thank you and goodbye. I wandered out into the sunshine feeling like something special had happened to me, and that people should notice. In a hospital, I suppose, everyone is special.

12th June

Went to lunch with a group of Colin's friends. I really resented the smokers in the group, especially the young ones. Here am I, trying to overcome a huge mental hurdle, recovering from two operations, and with radiation treatment and more surgery to come, and they are playing chicken with their lives. You can't even say they aren't aware of the risks – it's advertised enough nowadays. I felt like they were eating doughnuts in front of me while I was on a diet. I tried to explain this to Colin afterwards, but he pointed out that, in their defence, they weren't making a conscious effort to be offensive. I know this, but it doesn't make it any less hurtful.

I have given up drinking tea with almond milk in it. It tastes disgusting, and I'm sure herbal or lemon tea are healthier, anyway.

13th July

Struggling with my LID diet. The thing I miss is a real cup of tea. Nut milk is OK on cereals and in hot cocoa, but awful in tea. The bread is wonderful, and I bake a new loaf every day. It only lasts two days, and is then stale. It makes me think about how highly processed our food is, without us realising it.

Tissue scan today. Exactly the same as the bone scan, but picking up soft tissues instead of hard bones. Luckily, I only have to wait 30 minutes between the injection and the scan.

Amazingly, the doctor calls me into his office immediately after the scan, to discuss the results with me. I am grateful he does this, I am grateful he shows me the slides and explains them to me, I am grateful he treats me as an intelligent person and explains his findings. I find that I am grateful to all the hospital staff nowadays. I shall have to perfect a Uriah Heep accent to go with my new attitude. After all, my life does rest in the hands of these people.

The bone scan came back clear. Thank goodness for that. A cancer in the bone can't be cut out. They treat it with external beam radiation, but I suppose you are left with a weak bone forever.

Then he picks up the slides from this morning, and puts them on his light box. Two images of me – one from the front, and one from the back. He shows me the black blobs that indicate thyroid tissue activity. This could be healthy tissue that wasn't cut out by the surgeon, but there shouldn't be any thyroid tissue elsewhere in the body – if there is, it is probably cancerous. I stare at the screen. Not only are there strings of linked blobs up either side of my neck, but there is a blob under my right arm, too. The lymph nodes are infected. My mind immediately flies to the staging system – lymph node involvement is not too bad – 'distant metastases' (e.g. tumours in other parts of the body) are.

He feels my neck, to confirm the swollen lymph nodes. We discuss the fact that they will probably have to be cut out. I am not worried about the surgery in the way I was before – fear of the unknown giving rise to blind panic. I am worried about the pain afterwards. I don't tell him this, but nod sagely as if we are discussing garden design. He wonders about the armpit blob. An unusual location. He is reserving judgement until I have the CT scan. This won't be for another month. After that, he says, he should be able to discuss staging with me. I hate this waiting.

14th June

I have put on 4lb since being off my thyroid replacement medications. I'll be sorry to get the bloating that is sometimes a side effect of RAI. I have enough of that every month.

I looked up the effect of exposure to the sun on scar tissue. Opinions seem to vary, but general consensus seems to be to wear a sun-block for at least a year to give it time to heal properly. With all the worry, treatment, radiation and surgery going on, it seems surprising that this is so important to me. Ah, vanitas, vanitatum.

I am getting ready for the incarceration ahead of me. I am worried that I will panic when they hand me the pill, and make a scene.

15th June

Filled in a free prize draw entry today. When choosing my prize preference, I picked an immediate cash sum, rather than an annual income, like I usually do. I think it might represent better value.

I am beginning to feel the lack of thyroxine in my body. I feel like I have mumps, or that someone has their hands around my neck.

I came across a website today about thyroid cancer that suggested that a glow-in-the-dark Glow-worm doll would be an appropriate thing to take into hospital when you have your RAI. What a lovely idea. I have already thought about taking a teddy with me – I think we all revert a bit to childhood comforters in times of stress – and decided not to. I don't want him to get irradiated. What if it kills him? All my cuddly toys are safely put away on a shelf until I am safe again. I will treat them like I treat the pets.

I have found out that if you leave the water to cool a bit, you can have tea with almond or hazelnut milk! What a breakthrough! I should write a book. Or at the very least get on the telly.

16th June

My bag is packed with socks, slippers and extra sweatshirts. Everything can be machine-washed, so I can rinse it through when I get home. Who'd have thought radiation could be washed off? I can't get the images from Raymond Briggs' *When the Wind Blows* out of my mind.

The doctor rings to confirm my appointment, and tells me that he has looked again at the scan results, and is going to increase my radiation dose from 30 millicuries to 100 millicuries. He doesn't expand on his reasons, so I assume it's worse than he thought.

I ask about precautions when I come home from hospital. He tells me I can treat Colin as a 'carer', on the understanding that he will get some exposure to radiation, or like a member of the public. Hmm – hard choice – do I have an easy life and expose him to dangerous levels of radiation, or keep away from him for two weeks. Which option shall I choose? If I treat him like a member of the public, apparently I should use a separate bed for 17 days, before sleeping with him again. So I guess its OK to sleep with members of the public after that date, too.

I have considered the various ways of not being in the house at all while I am radioactive. Some people stay in a caravan in their garden. I don't have a caravan, but I have seriously considered camping out in the garage or in a tent, and only coming in to the house to use the loo, so that I am not near anyone. I decide that that would probably be going over the top. I don't know though - what price the health and safety of your family? Surely a few days discomfort is worth it? I decide to barricade myself in my bedroom, and prepare for a two-week siege. I check with Claire for the tenth time that she realizes she can't come near me when I come out of hospital. She rolls her eyes.

17th June

Three hours ago, they gave me 100 millicuries of radioactive iodine, and now I am confined to my room – a danger to society.

I have only just started to calm down now from the trauma of coming in here. When I arrived, I was shaking like a leaf, and in a huge panic. You know when you see people on the TV panic, and they can't think what to do? I was like that. The nurse rang to ask me to come in four hours early, and that completely threw me. I needed to wash my hair quickly, but half way through I forgot what to do! I was stood there dripping thinking - what next? I hadn't realised until then how frightened I had been. I had thought I was taking it all in my stride. Obviously my subconscious had different ideas.

The doctor brought the radioactive iodine to my room in a (presumably lead) carrier with a long handle. Reminded me of a spark plug spanner, but about the size of a beaker. He told me I was honoured to be offered it as a liquid instead of a pill, as a tribute to the speed with which this treatment had to be organised. He left the container inside the carrier, and put a straw in the top. He said it would taste like slightly stale water. It tasted like REALLY old water, which had been standing outside. For two weeks. With a plant and a dead beetle in it. He filled it up a couple of times with ordinary water, and got me to drink it down, to 'sloosh out' every little bit, and that was that. I was really worried about taking it, and worried that I'd make an embarrassing fuss. Luckily, I didn't. This is the sort of thing they should give out bravery awards for. Deliberately doing something that you know is dangerous is much braver than just living through things that happen to you.

Well, the door has been shut, the windows are sealed, and all the furniture is covered with plastic sheeting. Even the phone and television controller have been carefully taped up. The bin is marked with yellow tape showing the international 'radiation hazard' symbol. All this is an effort to make sure that none of my bodily fluids contaminate hospital property. I'll try not to sweat. The thermometer shows 27°, so it's not going to be easy.

Sitting here, I can hear the sounds of the nursing staff outside my room. The door has a little glass window cut into it, but I control the patterned pink curtain that spares me from prying eyes, making it less like a prison door peep-hole.

There are two daddy-long-legs and a fly in the room with me. I wonder if I can use them like canaries, and whether I should panic if they die?

I wonder what the reaction would be if I tried to leave? Who would be brave enough to stop me? How would they try? I imagine myself like The Incredible Hulk, raging through the corridors, while people shrink back, knocking into trolleys and sending crockery flying in their hurry to get as far away from me as possible. Shall I fling open the door, just to test the water?

A nurse pops in to see if I am OK. She pulls the door open a crack, shielding her body with the door, and talks with her head craned sideways. She tells me to buzz if I want anything. I think she secretly hopes I won't.

I ask for a tablet to ease the nausea, but whether it is caused by the radiation, the lack of sleep or the airless room, I don't know. Anyway, it works, and I sleep.

***

I have brought with me a store of healthy low-iodine snacks carefully packed in a supermarket 'Bag for Life'. I wonder who decides what a life-time should be? I'd like to know how long it will last, and who decided that this was the span of someone's years on this planet. A little old lady might be glad for twenty years of use, a young mother would want sixty or seventy. Can a supermarket really guarantee their scheme will last this long? Can you sue them if it doesn't? My bag already has a split in it and lists sadly sideways. Somehow I would feel I was letting it down by trading it in. You wouldn't trade in a person, would you?

A stunted sapling tree stretches up towards the sky, the side towards my window dead and lifeless, leaves only showing on the furthest branches. Does it too want to get afar away as possible from the contamination?

OK. Time to snap out of the pathos. I shall be expecting Ryan O'Neal to come and lay on the bed beside me at this rate. Being on your own gets you like that. The mind moves in places it doesn't usually go – released from the usual tasks of organising daily life. Perhaps that's why a lot of great artists were invalids. Only they had the time to devote to 'higher things'. What if Keats had been perfectly healthy, or Coleridge not addicted? If Virginia Woolfe had taken a job, or Jane Austen married, would the world be a poorer place?

I feel like a heroine in a Jean Plaidy novel – Mary Queen of Scots maybe – shut up with nothing to do but record her thoughts. No contact with the outside world. No visitors allowed. This morning I was terrified – sick and shaking. Now I am just bored.

The shower in here emits such a hugely powerful blast of water, I feel like an elephant being hosed down. I imagine blobs of radioactive liquid mingling with waste-water,floating like dollops of oil. It reminds me of the opening sequence of The Simpsons.

Into bed early for eight hours of sweating and dribbling myself free of this poison. The nurse brings me another anti-nausea tablet.

18th June

I lie on my bed, tracing the patterns of painted jasmine and honeysuckle across the ceiling. Outside the window, there are no plants. Only tumbled cobbles and a sun-streaked mural that has seen better days. Ivy is pushing its way through a crack in the plaster-work – one day it will be everywhere. If I was feeling particularly morbid, I would compare it to a cancer, insidiously inching (centimetre-ing?) its way into the very fabric of its host, digging its tendrils in, and destroying that which supports it. At least cancer dies with its host, and cannot continue. Unchecked, ivy can cover a whole forest.

I take another shower. I don't feel so sick today, although I was cold in the night, even at this constant temperature. The nurse brought me an extra blanket.

I am feeling stifled in here. I keep changing the lights from main light to side lights, and stay as near the window as I can, to make use of the natural light. One thing I will remember next time is an aerosol air freshener. I try jogging on the spot to perk up my system, and it works for a while. I am worried the nurse will come and ask what I am doing. Oh well.

Colin visited me this afternoon! He was allowed 15 minutes, standing at the door, with me on the other side of the room. It felt odd not to be able to touch him, but it really lifted my spirits.

I am feeling rather sick again today. When lunch comes, I scrape it down the toilet, flushing twice as instructed. Anyone monitoring what comes out probably wouldn't be able to tell that it hadn't already been through me. I feel like a naughty child. I eat hazelnuts and dried apples instead.

I have a look for my canary-flies, and can't find them. I hope they have escaped.

The skin on my legs, arms and face is peeling. The Vitamin E cream I have been using on my scar is wonderful – thick and creamy. It mixes with the flaky bits and forms a thin layer of skin porridge.

I get a visit from the nuclear physics department, who tell me that they have been charting my progress with a Geiger counter in the ceiling. They can tell when I leave the main room to go into the bathroom, and see how the levels of radiation have fallen when I return. They think I can go home tomorrow.

I am put back on my triiothyronine.

June 19th

Up early, jet-washed, packed and ready to go by 8.30am.

I know I am ill, but I don't really feel like it. I've felt worse than this after a hard night out! I suppose I would feel ill if the cancer really gets hold. I wonder what it would (will?) feel like. Would you slowly get weaker, and sink gracefully into oblivion, or would bits of you stop working, like a death from diabetes? I don't think death is that easy.

The radiation should now have done its job and I need to flush it out as quickly as possible. I drink glass after glass of room-temperature water – remember that's 27°!

The health and safety man has been and given me a pep-talk about safety measures. These are to protect people with functioning thyroid glands from the radiation. Most at risk are small children and pregnant women. He advises me not to stay in public places for longer than an hour at a time. This means, for example, that I can go shopping, but not to the cinema. I am not to exceed one hour's exposure at close quarters with any adult, or more than a few minutes with a child. He hands me a small, folded card which looks like a war-time ration book. I think someone over-ordered in about 1948. I hope they got a good deal for bulk purchasing. I am to carry this card with me everywhere I go, and follow the instructions until 7th July.

He tells me there is a Geiger counter in the roof of my room, so they could monitor me from their office. They said when I went to the (en-suite) toilet, they could tell I was out of the main room, and when I came back, the level was lower where'd I'd flushed some of it down the toilet. Shades of Big Brother.

Still feeling sick. I think it is the lack of thyroxine. Sea sickness tablets sort it out.

I heard someone on the television today saying how it helped her to come to terms with her breast cancer by having it written down. Her secretary friend attended her doctor's appointments with her and took down the in formation in shorthand. What a good idea – you can never assimilate the information in one go.

20th June

Spent a restless night on a pillow covered with plastic carrier bags (under the pillowcase). A bit noisy! I have woken up feeling sick and tired. Wondering how to get through the day avoiding mothers with children and not being in the same room with Colin for more than an hour. I am hoping it will get easier as I go along. Every time I blow my nose, I rush to the bathroom to throw the tissue down, and flush it away. I eat delicately off my fork at mealtimes, trying not to get spit on it. I use plastic spoons that can be thrown away.

My food is beginning to taste funny. Or rather, NOT to taste funny – in fact, it is beginning to not taste of anything at all.

I emailed a friend who has thyroid cancer, telling her about the little card they had issued. She wrote back:

> *Ha, I got that little war time card too! No, I didn't carry it round with me. Didn't think I needed to. As long as you don't attempt to fly, and set off any radio-active sensor alarms, you should be ok! I was told to stay away from the dentist and hairdressers for 3 weeks. I've decided to keep these cards - I'm not sure why.*
> *Kathy*

I am going to keep my card too. I think it is because it is a concrete reminder of something that will otherwise get pushed to the back of the mind and forgotten. It's like a war medal. We can use it to prove we did something unusual and brave.

21st June

I am beginning to feel quite ill now that I have been off they thyroxin for over a week. That makes it all the more difficult to concentrate on the safety of my family. If it was because I didn't want them to catch my cold, for example, that would be OK – the pressure wouldn't be there. It is SO IMPORTANT that they don't stay in the room with me, or eat from the same cutlery, in case they are permanently damaged. It doesn't make it easier that they are blasé about it – Claire can't see far enough into the future to appreciate the effects it could have, and Colin is just selflessly brave. I have made him go and stay in a different house so that the pressure is not on me to stay away from him.

I refused to give Claire a lift in the car this morning, and she thinks I am being deliberately horrible to her. I am having to concentrate really hard on using a separate towel, throwing my used tissues down the toilet, washing up my dishes separately. Only another day, and I think I can relax a bit. I'll still have to keep away from Claire.

Wrote an email to an old friend, saying that I had been diagnosed with cancer last month. It seems incredible that it is only that long ago. I know it is a cliché, but it feels like a lifetime. I suppose that is the thing with clichés, they make sense, because they are so often true.

Feeling sorry for myself. I may start reading Keats and laying on the sofa……

22nd June

Had another argument with Claire about her going out too much. She pointed out that I wanted her out of the way so that she didn't get irradiated. I couldn't argue with that.

I am so stressed by washing and cleaning everything. I will be glad when it is over. I wish I had cling-filmed the door handles, and phone, but I think it is too late now. In two weeks time, I will put my (undoubtedly dribbled-on) pillow in the garage for two weeks to 'cool down'. The timings are so inexact; everyone gives different lengths of time.

Two things I have realised are 1. how often I put my fingers in my mouth, and 2.how much my eyes water in the mornings! I have worn a path to the bathroom by my constant need to go there to either wash my hands or throw a tissue down the loo.

Got this email from a friend:

> *Keep on smiling – it's good therapy, and at least you still have your own teeth!*
> *Joan*

It's these little messages that keep me going!

23rd June

I am really feeling the strain of constantly being on my guard every time I move. I am feeling a lot better now, but the effects of being hypothyroid (not having enough thyroid hormone in my blood) are still showing. I am cold, and very forgetful – I can go into a room and forget why I am there several times in a row. I am also very clumsy, and keep dropping things, and knocking into stuff. Bit like PMT.

I had a chat with Claire today. She is very worried, both about the possibility of my dying, and about the effects exposure to my radiation might have on her. I have tried to put her mind at rest, while still frightening her enough to make her stay careful for another few days. Not easy! I am very worried about contaminating her, obviously, and cannot reassure her, as she would like. I am glad she is talking to me now. We have discussed the fact the thyroid cancer is very slow-growing, but I have been honest with her, and told her that the doctor still hasn't done enough tests to tell me what he thinks about a prognosis. I hope to know within the next 4-6 weeks. It is so difficult to wait – we are used to doctors dealing with specifics, or at least seeming to.

Went to the hospital for yet another scan today. Sat as far away from everybody in the waiting room as I could, and got out as soon as I had finished. I am used to them now, and close my eyes, think of England, and wait until they are done. It makes a big difference when you have a radiologist who explains the procedure to you, and talks you through it. Didn't look like there was much take-up, but I suppose that develops later. Or perhaps it means that it's all gone!

24th June

I am feeling a lot better now. I think there is only so long you can go on being melancholy. Having had the RAI, and knowing I am being treated has been a big boost, although I know there is lots more to come yet.

I now feel I can look to the future, and plan things to do. Previously, I had been in a big fluffy cloud, unable to see two feet in front of me. The clichés about swimming in treacle, and pushing through cotton wool are all spot on. Coming to terms with the cancer has taken over my life. It was something that I needed to work through before moving on. People say it's like a grieving process, and I can see what they mean. Suddenly nothing makes sense. Your whole life has to be re-evaluated against a different set of standards. Of course, once this has been done, you can file it and move on. I am (happily) now in this position. One more cliché – I feel like a great weight has been lifted off my mind. It was like struggling with a mathematical equation for weeks on end, and now I have suddenly found the answer. I can put it to one side, and sort out all the other stuff that has been stacking up waiting to be dealt with.

I am still washing my clothes out every day.

25th June

Going by the calculations recommended by the Imperial Cancer Research Health and Safety Department, I think that I am over the worst part now. The only really contaminated part of me now is my saliva. I still feel really tired, and am having a nap every afternoon. At last, though, I feel that I am coming out of it.

Someone from the internet support group wrote:

> *I think the solitary confinement and feeling like a leper are the things that made me feel crazy. Marybeth*

And she's right. It's not the feeling ill bit. We've all been ill at some point in our lives, and I can live with that. It's the feeling of being so totally alone, and the lack of human contact that bring you down.

26th June

Starting to make plans to continue with my life. I have been reviewing the staging systems again, and trying to make a prediction. I have also been looking at some stories of people with advanced thyroid cancer, and seen how much worse their cases are than mine. I am lucky to have no bone metastases, and nothing showing in my lungs. I am unlucky to have cancer in my lymph nodes, but this shouldn't affect my survival, although it may affect the possibility of the cancer coming back again. All in all, I think I have probably got off quite lightly. I think I will wait a few more weeks until the doctor confirms this, and then take it from there. I read today that although thyroid cancer has previously been considered a life-long disease, many doctors now think that if you have not had a recurrence in 10 years, you can consider yourself clear – what a great thought!

27th June

My 44th birthday. I can go out to dinner as long as I can eat it in 59 minutes.

I am planning to go back to work next week, as soon as I am no longer a public danger! It'll be odd to go back and carry on as though nothing had happened. In a way, I am keen to put it behind me, but I am also keen to get it sorted out, so I can start again with a 'clean slate'. I don't want it hanging over me. I am frightened of brushing it off as a minor inconvenience, and finding out I am going to die. I think I should be reading about the disease, and fighting it somehow, not simply carrying on regardless. I think I will look up cancer-prevention diet recommendations.

I have stripped the bed again today, and washed the bed linen and under-blanket as before. The duvet and pillows have gone into the loft until next winter – should be un-radiated by then - and I am using the spare set. I have to have more radiation treatment in November, and I will change over the duvets again after that. How lucky that I am having my treatments just in time to swop from summer to winter duvets!

28th June

I still haven't got my taste back since the RAI. Everything tastes like sunflower oil, with an odd metallic twang to it. I gather this is a common side-effect of RAI, and that it can take anything from a few weeks to a few months for it to get back to normal.

I am still being very careful about anything to do with my mucus-y bodily fluids (eg wiping my nose, licking things), but I'm not being so vigilant about other things, such as washing my hands all the time in case I have sweaty palms.

29th June

Every day I move forward, and make some progress towards getting my life back to normal. I have another week of keeping away from people, and then I should be almost back to normal. I am still very tired, and trying to do the things I used to do is rather a strain. I think this is because of being inactive for so long due to the two operations, as well as to the RAI.

Logged into the internet support group this afternoon, and took comfort from being able to answer other people's questions. The most worrisome ones are often about seemingly trivial issues. The sillier the question, the harder it is to ask, sometimes, but they are usually the most worrisome ones. I asked how everyone else managed to continue their lives and fit all the treatments in, too.

I got this reply:

> *Take it a step at a time. Ask for help with the big stuff and let the small stuff go. You will be fine!*
> *Best wishes,*
> *Ellen, Phoenix AZ.*

30th June

Every day in every way I am getting better and better. Who was it recommended that you start every day repeating that phrase? I don't know if it works as a cure, but it is certainly how I feel at the moment. It is amazing that in less that two months I have gone through so many emotions.

I have now come to accept that I have cancer, that it will be treated, and that I can't do anything about finding a foolproof projected life-span. I don't know if spending so much time researching thyroid cancer helped me come to this decision, but it certainly helped me at the time. It helped me to understand what was going on, so that I was not left wondering all the time. It makes me much more able to understand what the doctors say to me, and to take in the in formation at the meetings I have. Somehow treatment is not so worrying when you understand what is happening and why.

It also helps a great deal to know the possible risks of any treatment. Even if the risks are high, at least they have a limit – if you do not know, you imagine all sorts of things.

July – a month of butterflies and buddleia. Hot summer days, and a chill in the heart.

1st July

Almost everybody knows someone who has or who has had cancer. Is the statistic one in three of us? That's an awful lot.

I am still very tired, and feel like I need a rest every afternoon. By the time it gets to 2.30pm, my legs feel like they are ready to collapse under me. I don't know how much longer this will go on, or why it is happening. Is it because of the operations? Is it because of the radiation treatment? Is it because of the stress? I wish I knew whether it was because I am weak through lack of exercise and need to work my body harder, or whether it is because my body is completely worn out and needs to rest. I think I'll try to be more active in the mornings, and make sure I have at least an hour's rest in the afternoon, with my feet up. If I fall asleep, it must be because my body needs it. Having a nap in the afternoon doesn't seem to be affecting the amount of sleep I need at night.

2nd July

I am still waking up in the night, and have been since the RAI. I don't know whether it is a side-effect of the treatment, or just stress because of being ill.

I have arranged to go back to work next week, mornings only at first. I feel very guilty about the amount of time I am having off – I have been off for three months now, and am going to have to have two more blocks for four weeks off before Christmas. How unfair on employers to have to cover this. Although I know it is my right to have this time off, I am very grateful to them for being sympathetic.

3rd July

Bob and Julia came round today. They were very wary of being close to me, because of the radiation, even though I am so close to my 'release date'. I think that younger people are more able to accept radiation as A Good Thing, whereas people brought up through the CND, Ban the Bomb, women at Greenham Common era still think of it as the big mistake of the twentieth century. And perhaps we are right.

I have been looking again at the prognosis chart. I wish the doctor would hurry up and tell me what his opinion is! I am really tempted to follow the argument that I can't do anything about it, so I might as well ignore the problem and get on with my life. But what if I have a limited lifespan and don't do anything about it? What if I fritter away my few remaining years until I start to be too ill to do anything about it? Or is the danger that I will spend so long worrying about it that I still won't get time to do anything, and will be ill from stress-related illnesses as well! Who knows? Would it be easier if we had all the answers? Or would it take away the excitement of life? What if we all had a specific allotted life-span, and knew the day we were going to die? Would you use your life any more wisely? Probably not.

4th July

I am beginning to go a bit 'stir crazy' cooped up in the house all the time. It is all beginning to look beautifully clean and tidy, like a show home, but no-one ever comes, and I never go out. My friends work all day, and the only people I ever talk to are the checkout staff at the supermarkets, and the double glazing salesmen who ring. I shall be very glad to get back to work. I feel like my mind is beginning to go. I don't know whether its because of the constant tiredness I now feel, or whether its lack of use. I keep forgetting things. The thyroxin must have kicked in by now, so I don't think it's that.

5th July

I still haven't got my taste back. I am going to put weight back on again soon if I keep eating like I am at the moment. The lack of taste is making food seem bland and unpalatable, and because of this I keep leaving things half-finished and trying something else instead. I feel I need something nice to eat as a treat, and when something doesn't satisfy me, I just try something else. Alcohol seems to do the trick...

6th July

Someone asked me today whether having cancer has changed the way I look at my life. It hasn't. I still have the same responsibilities as any mother. I still have to go to work every day to earn a living. I still have the housework to do. So I haven't planned the vacation of a lifetime, and I'm not thinking about selling up and moving to the country – although that would be nice! It hasn't made me want to run my life any differently at all. I would like to say that it has made me want to live for the day, and throw caution to the wind, but that isn't the case. I am too sensible for that.

I am hoping that the doctor will tell me soon what my prognosis is. Perhaps what he tells me will alter my view of life. I wonder what I would do if he said I had only five or ten years to live. What if he said I wasn't likely to see my sixtieth birthday? Would I spend spend spend? Or would I want to keep everything as normal as possible for as long as possible? I don't think I'd spend all my money, because that's part of Claire's inheritance. Also, I might find that I need my money to spend on nursing me at the end of my life. How annoyed I'd be if I couldn't get out of bed with out help, but that I'd spent all my money on a luxury cruise and couldn't afford help. These are questions that you can never answer until you are in that position. You can speculate as often and as deeply as you like, but you can never really KNOW until the time comes.

7th July

Free of restrictions at last! I can now go out and spit on people, and sneeze in public places! I have worried so much about my family, and I know that they have been worried too. It has been quite a stressful time for me, worrying about almost every move I made, and concentrating on things that normally done unconsciously. I have learnt some useful things, like wetting my fingers at the tap when I want to open a plastic bin bag, and how to flip the pages of a book over with dry hands. All very sanitary, and things I should have learnt a long time ago, I am sure.

8th July

This morning I had a CT scan. I got a very nice letter explaining what would happen to me. It was very much the same as the other scans – injection, then being fed under a star-gate shaped machine. It took twenty minutes. They did one of my neck, and one of my chest, presumably to see if I have any tumours in my lungs. I am getting very blasé about it all now. Someone told me that a PET/CT scan in the USA cost her $1,000. Hurrah for the NHS. How would I have managed if I had had to pay for it all? I suppose if that were the system we'd all have insurance. Still, a sobering thought.

I am going back to work tomorrow, and am now intent on planning the summer holidays. I am going to ignore the fact that I have more treatment coming up, and live as I did before. I still have it in the back of my mind that I need to go into hospital again, but I am not going to let it rule my life. I feel well, and until I feel ill again, I am not going to let anything worry me.

I thought I would be worried about knowing that I had cancer growing inside me. When I first learnt that the thyroid gland they cut out of my neck had contained cancer cells, I was very glad that it was all gone, and I was able to say that I had had cancer, but no longer did. When I found out there was cancer in the lymph glands, I was really still too ill and depressed to take much notice. It seemed like one more nail in the coffin. Now I have come out of that depression, I find it odd that I have this growing inside of me, and yet it doesn't affect my life. Perhaps it's because I can't see it, that it doesn't affect me. I can actually feel one of the lumps, and I get little pin-pricks of pain now and then, but perhaps these are psychosomatic. Some of it will already be dying because it has been killed by the RAI. I think I will be glad when it is gone.

It is two months ago today that I found out I had cancer.

9th July

I feel quite good today. I have been reading Gone With the Wind, and think that what I have been through isn't so bad after all. Looking forward to the rest of the summer now.

10th July

Shared my experiences with a girl who has recently been diagnosed with thyroid cancer (or thyca, as we initiates call it).

She wrote back:

> *Sue,*
>
> *I can't tell you how much your note has helped me. It has given me hope! Let's stay in touch. I'd like to know how you're doing as things progress.*
>
> *All the best, Michele*

Perhaps I can be the next Deanna Troy, counsellor extraordinaire. I'll have to grow my hair a bit, and work on my legs.

11th July

Half day at work today. How very odd. Of course, a lot of people I don't work with didn't even realise I'd been gone. But a lot did. I don't think I've ever been hugged so much in my life! Certainly not in the workplace. (No, not even at the Christmas party). Everyone was very, very nice, and said they were glad I was back. Aahhh…

12th July

Phone call from my uncle today. This is someone who phones about once every five years, so that shows what an impact my illness has had on the family. We are hardly ever ill. In fact, I can't really remember anyone being ill at all. Only when we are going to die.

13th July

Sunny today. Have been in the garden, trying to catch up with everything. Poor plants look very sorry for themselves. Never mind, a nice lot of weeding has filled up the compost heap, so they'll have loads to eat next year.

14th July

Went to work as usual this morning, and the consultant's secretary rang to ask me to come in straight away. I suggested 2pm, and she asked me if I could make it any earlier. I stupidly thought he has double booked, and thought no more about it.

At the meeting, I was told that my cancer is poorly differentiated. This means that it doesn't take up radioactive iodine like it should, and therefore hasn't been killed off. The consultant wants me to go to London to be operated on by a specialist surgeon in St Thomas' Hospital, who will surgically remove the remaining bits. I was quite stunned by this. I sat there and smiled, while my mind kept still. It felt like I was trying to drive a car over a kerbstone or out of a muddy rut. My brain was revving and revving, but not going anywhere. Even when he said that the surgeon might have to break my breastbone to get to the cancer, I smiled and said OK. In this situation, one has to agree.

He is also going to give me more radioactive iodine afterwards. I am not sure why. I think he thinks I might take it up better a second time. I wasn't really listening by this stage. He thought I was worried about the surgery - I am worried because I have Hashimoto's thyroiditus (when your body produces thyroid antibodies), and am resistant to RAI, so they won't know I have it in the first place (because it makes the tests unreliable), and when they do, they won't be able to treat it. Now this IS a scary bit. I have a complete and utter faith in the medical profession (providing you keep an eye on them). But what happens when the tools at their disposal don't work? What then?

I am booked in to go to London tomorrow, and he has given me all my notes and x-rays in a large plain brown envelope. I feel a bit like a spy, for some reason. I certainly feel that it's something I shouldn't be leaving the hospital with. Colin drives me home.

15th July

Up to St Thomas' today. Sat on the train in a bit of a daze. I felt like James Stewart, unexpectedly finding myself in a black-and-white movie. After sitting with the x-rays on my lap for a while, looking furtive, I balanced them on the parcel rack. It all seemed rather bizarre and other-worldly. No-one challenged me, though, and we arrived safely.

Very nice surgeon. Put me completely at ease. He was rather surprised at how much thyroid tissue was left in my neck, and thinks that might be the reason for the poor RAI uptake. So that's OK then.

He told me that the pin-pricks of feeling I have been having in my neck are the nerves knitting back together after the surgery. It's nice to know that I'm not going completely mad, and that it isn't all in my mind. And it's also nice to know that my neck is on the mend, however slowly it's going.

Booked in for the day after he comes back from his holidays. When I checked on the Internet, it says that waiting time for this particular surgeon is 226 days. Am I honoured, or seriously ill? It certainly brings it home to you how ill you are, when you are put to the front of the queue like that.

16th July

The good news is that I feel better than I have for 15-20 years now that they have cut a large lump of cancer out of me, and I am bounding with energy. I don't mind the surgery, as long as I feel this good in between. Worked all day, and what's more, I thoroughly enjoyed it!

17th July

Sat in the garden this morning and read my book. Well, what a waste of summer it has been staying out of the sun if I am going to have it all done again. All those days lost. All that tanning time wasted. Here I am, all pasty and white, while everyone else has a healthy golden glow. Oh well, chalk '1' up in the 'avoidance of skin cancer' column.

18th July

Sitting in the garden watching the butterflies on the buddleia bushes, I wonder about their short lives. Am I right in thinking they only live for one day? Or is that dragonflies? How short a time to do everything that you have to do. But then again, if they are anything like us, they waste it all, flittering about from one luscious drooping bloom to another, sipping the nectar, sunning their wings, looking for love, and then suddenly it's all over. One day you look behind, ten years have gone, you find. Or twenty, or thirty. You missed the starting gun, and no-one told you when to run. You find your body is unable to do the things you want it to, you have notched up responsibilities that you can't leave, and gradually your inclination to change the world seeps away. Perhaps someone else will start the things you wished you'd done, and make the world a better place. Dream on.

19th July

Drinks and nibbles at Bob and Julia's. Lots of lovely people I know asking me how I am, and, most refreshingly, lots of lovely people I don't know, who talk to me about other things altogether. It makes me feel like a real person again, and not merely the sum of my various treatments and scars.

20th July

I've been out in the garden today, looking at all the flowers and plants growing. What I like best are the new shoots pushing their way up through the earth. I've always liked that. That is why spring is my favourite season, with the sharp points of bulb leaves poking their way up through the frost. It always gives me hope in the future, and makes me thing that all things are possible. If a little leaf can push its way through the icy ground, then what isn't possible?

21st July

I've been looking back over this diary. You can tell which days I've had nothing to do, can't you? For all those days in isolation in RAI, the pages are long. I wonder if you could match up the days with most writing against the sunny days of the year?

I'm sure the weather has a lot to do with my mood, and when I am happy, I write less because I'm off doing stuff.

22nd July

My life is on hold at the moment. I have been talking to a Julie about what she has planned for the rest of the summer, and I have realised that I can't plan anything, and haven't been able to do so for months. I can't plan a holiday, or an exhibition, or a visit, or anything. I don't know when I will be in hospital, or when I'll be too ill to do things. I might be perfectly well at any given time, but I don't know. I have to leave my calendar blank until further notice. I have been invited to a wedding, and don't know if I'll be able to go. I wonder when I'll be able to plan stuff again? Will I be well by Christmas? Will I not be well again until next summer? I hope they tell me soon.

23rd July

Having thought yesterday that I can't plan anything, I have decided that I can't let my whole life be ruled by 'what ifs'. I have ordered a new kitchen. If I wait until I am well, then I might not have a new one for another year. I have ordered it, and if it has to stay in the garage until I am well enough to help put it together, then so be it. I have taken control of my life again. Hurrah!

24th July

Started booking things into my life with a vengeance. I have decided that it's no use sitting around and waiting for the next bit of treatment. If I do that, I could waste months. I must try and fill up the bits in between as best I can. If I have to cancel things, then that's just hard luck. So I am now down to do two exhibitions, three visits and a dinner party.

25th July

Sat in the garden, reading my book, looking at the pretty flowers, watching the butterflies, and thinking how lucky I am to get sick pay. Even from depths of great trauma, I can think happy thoughts, and generate a spark of optimism. Gotta be good!

26th July

I think I am getting sorted out. I am gradually getting things back in place. Putting things back where they belong in my life. I don't mean tidying up cupboards, although this is part of it. What I mean is, that I am psychologically tying up loose ends. I am trying to finish projects that I have started, and get my life into some sort of order.

Once I have done this, I will be able to start again. I need a blank sheet to work on, a straight line to go on from. The last few months, things have been all put out of place. I understand now what people mean when they say their lives are 'torn apart'. Things don't seem to follow in the same order, time moves erratically, and the activities which once gave structure to our days suddenly stop supporting us. It takes time to re-organise a whole lifestyle. Old habits have to be re-learnt. This is the time to make decisions on what to keep and what to throw away. And, ironically, this is the very time that you can't make in formed decisions. Things often get done because you don't care very much any more what happens. Give us time. Give us space. That disorientated feeling will hopefully pass, and life will begin again.

27th July

Spoke to Helen, who had thyroid cancer some years ago. She talked to me about how my priorities in life will change once I get over the treatment and have time to sit and take stock of things. I don't know. I don't feel very different at the moment.

28th July

I have been thinking about what Helen said yesterday. Perhaps I should take a different outlook on life, now my perceived future has changed so much. Or has it? If I'd been given a definite life-span (shortened or otherwise), I think it would be different. I'd be able to think and plan. As everything is still so vague, I'm finding it hard to see anything in between everything staying the same, and dying in a few short years. I suppose I am beginning to think about what I want to do with the time I have left more seriously than before. I certainly think more about taking responsibility for my own healthcare.

29th July

Peeled all the labels off the LID food today. Thank goodness. My kitchen now looks a lot neater and tidier. Hopefully I won't need them again. Of course, going through the cupboards did make me realise how dirty everything is. Another job on the list.

30th July

Nothing of note happened at all today. Just a bit of housework, and some cooking. Read a few chapters of my book, and played on the computer for a while. Idyllic or boring?

31st July

For several days in a row, I have forgotten to take my tablets in the morning. When they were first prescribed, it was all new and exciting, and I made a special effort to remember. Now it's every day, it seems not so important somehow. I am sure that in time, I'll pass this phase, and make it part of my daily routine. Hope so!

August – a month of seagulls and shells. Once more into the breach, dear friends …

1st August

Took an art exhibition down today. I was able to join in almost as if I was a normal person. That will soon all change again. I hate the fact that this treatment is all so spaced out, and I have so little time in between to do the things I want to do. I suppose I should be pleased that I have any time at all, really.

In a way, I think I would rather be really ill, but for a shorter time, than be in this constant state of convalescence. I am wasting my life away just resting.

2nd August

Despite what I said yesterday, I am still not strong. My poor muscles have got months of inactivity to catch up on before I am back to my old self again. I will avoid going into the garage for a while; it upsets me too much to see it in that state. I'll stay indoors and do a little light dusting instead.

3rd August

Bought a pill dispenser today. Very useful. I don't have a problem taking the tablets, but I do have problems remembering whether or not I have taken them, later in the day. This handy little gadget has solved all that. Three cheers for the modern inventor.

4th August

Saw my consultant again today. Nothing of note to report. I am so used to going into hospitals now that I swan in and out as if I work there. I think I should be given a red badge or something similar to identify me as a regular user. They took more blood.

One thing I did find out today, was how fast the internal grapevine system works in that particular department. I made a smart remark to the receptionist as I sat in the waiting room, and by the time I met the nurse who was doing the blood letting, she'd heard all about it! Wow!

5th August

Went to the dentist today, and complained of toothache. I told him my recent medical history, as instructed, and he said he wouldn't do anything else to me, and to come back in six months time. In the meantime, I'll have to chew on one side only.

6th August

We were discussing self-portraits today, and a recent exhibition of before-and-after portraits of cosmetic surgery patients. Without thinking about it, I said that if I did a self-portrait, it would have great red lines coming out of the neck, like an explosion. Quite odd, the way this image came into my mind. A moment of artistic inspiration I didn't know I felt that strongly about having the cancer. How odd to get a flash of insight into your own subconscious mind.

7th August

Worked seriously on my booklet on radioiodine treatment and the low iodine diet today. Made me feel like a real writer, sitting here tapping away at the keys. Perhaps I could be the next Enid Blyton. Did she write booklets about cancer? I think not.

8th August

My new kitchen arrived today. Goodness knows when I will be able to sort it out, let alone put it up. I asked the delivery men to stack it neatly in the garage. I don't think it will get put in for a very long time.

9th August

Struggling to catch up on my life now. I have missed more than half of the summer. Everyone else is going around looking tanned and beautiful, and I am white and flabby. If only I could get into my garage to reach the skiing machine, I'd be OK, but there's a kitchen stacked in front of it. If I moved the things out of the present kitchen, there would be room in there. But where would the things I take out be stored? Moving things around in my head, I realise that the first thing on the list is clearing out the cupboard under the stairs. I decide to do some gardening instead. There's always something soothing about pottering around in the sun, poking at the plants, seeing what's growing, smelling the earth. I like to walk around in bare feet, feeling the ground beneath me. I don't know if that gives a deep psychological insight into the state of my mental health, or if it means that I haven't got many pairs of shoes.

10th August

Trying to get to grips with cleaning the house. It has been left for so long now. There is only so many times you can ask someone to come in and help you 'do'. I need a lady who 'does'. Permanently! Perhaps if I paint over it all, I won't have to clean it? Tidying up seems to take all my time, let alone cleaning what's underneath. I have never really recovered from moving house six weeks before and my things have never been allocated a proper place. Hence, they all seem to be roaming the house under their own steam, moving from location to location. Nothing is ever anywhere you expect it to be.

11th August

I am a lot better to day. Really as if I am getting my health back. Which is ironic, as I now have to go back into hospital for a major operation. I think getting the house sorted out has helped a lot. It feels a lot more calming when it is clean and tidy. Good for the soul.

12th August

Trying to sort out Claire's school uniform today, as I don't think I will be in a fit state to do it after my surgery. When I go into shops and buy back-to-school pencil cases etc, everyone must think I am Mrs Super-organised. I ordered school shirts off the Internet. I am getting good at that now.

13th August

My freezer is getting packed with goodies. I'd like to say 'with home-made goodies', but I never was much good at lying. Good old Tesco's has helped out again.

14th August

Hooray! My reimbursed travel costs arrived today. There's a little ray of sunshine in the darkness of this whole encounter! It's an expensive business going to and from hospitals on an almost weekly basis. Each trip costs me £5.

15th August

Crying again today. I have been working hard on the house, and trying not to think about going into hospital, but I think that perhaps that hasn't been the best thing. I should have moaned to everyone and got it out of my system. Isn't that what counselling is all about? Well, this is a cheaper way of doing it. Just costs a lot in paper tissues. Started to pack.

16th August

My ex-sister-in-law died today. I didn't expect to feel so shocked. I cried (again) quite a lot. I suppose I should be quantifying/qualifying this crying I keep referring to. Sometimes it comes out as a bit of a grizzle, but more often than not, it's huge uncontrollable sobs of complete

blackness and despair. I think if I read through this, I would realise that I have only mentioned the worst cases. I cry so much now, it's not really worth putting it down each time. I think the phrase 'crying as if my heart would break' sums it up. If I am standing up, I have to sit down, and it's not beautiful, trickling-tears crying, it's open-mouthed, dribbling-from-every-orifice-on-the-face crying. Not a pretty sight.

Anyway, I was told she'd died today, and it made me realise how awful dying is. No more contact ever again with the people you have known. I am glad I am fighting my own battle as best I know how. I don't have a long list of 'things I want to do before I die', but I would like to have the opportunity to do things if I do ever want to.

17th August

Sorted out the last few things before being out of commission for two weeks (allowing for recuperation). What a lot to do! I have left little notes, again, for Claire and Colin, but I don't know if they will ever get read.

18th August

Went to stay at my parent's house overnight, as they live closer to London than I do. They are remarkably calm, and we talked about everything but the operation. Are they in denial? Or kindly trying to keep it low-key? Took my mind off it, anyway, It is so nice to be out of my normal surroundings.

19th August

What a different hospital! Everyone is so nice! I don't mean to be horrid about the other hospital I went into, but this one is so much better! Is it because it serves the affluent capital?

The anaesthetist came, and talked to me about putting a tube down my throat. I must have looked horrified, because she quickly back-tracked and offered me a face-mask instead.

Got sliced and diced, and am out with relatively little pain. I think the anaesthetic still hasn't worn off. I have got two drain tubes in my neck, pinning me to the bed, as before, a drip for fluids in the back of my hand, and a drip for morphine, too. I press the button when I need pain relief. I also have one of those clear plastic tubes that they are so fond of on TV hospital programmes. I now realise that they don't go up your nose at all. The tube clips onto the front of your nose, like a false moustache, and has a tiny hole in it, where the oxygen comes out. The surgeon hasn't put padding over my neck, and I can feel little 'bobbles'. The nurse tells me that the three incisions are held together with temporary thread, and the ends are secured with little beads. They call it my pearl necklace.

When I wanted to go to the toilet this afternoon, they tried to make me use a bedpan. Ha! No chance! I tried, but couldn't do it, and made them bring me a commode. Bit of a struggle moving all the tubes, and they weren't keen on disconnecting the oxygen. I convinced them that three minutes off it wasn't going to do me any harm, as it was just a belt-and-braces thing.

20th August

I have a lovely electric bed that goes up and down top, sides, middle and bottom. I think it even makes the tea if you ask it nicely.

An old friend who lives in London came to visit me today, and it was good to catch up on all the news. Judging from my last operations, I must have looked awful. A big, fat, fluff, bloated grey face, with about six double chins, I guess. I haven't actually looked in a mirror yet. Time for that later, when I am feeling stronger.

21st August

Good thing that happened today: managed to get dressed. The nurse said I was a very determined lady.

Bad thing that happened today: they took away my bed! I needed it after the operation to help me sleep upright, (and still feel as if I need it, actually), but someone has just come out of surgery, and is more deserving, so I get to play with piles of pillows instead.

Nice view from the window, down the Thames. I can look out at all the scurrying people, and the red London buses. There is a market stall selling tourist knick-knacks on the embankment. Whenever I look out, it always seems to be surrounded by customers (or browsers). Perhaps I should change jobs when I get out?

There is a homeless person who stays for the night in the hospital garden, wrapped in his sleeping bag, hidden from people at ground level behind the bushes. At least I can see the end to my troubles.

22nd August

Home today. What a trauma. My legs are still wobbly, so I feel like Bambi when I walk. I look awful, with a cut neck and steri-strips all over my neck. My face is grey, and my hair is sticking up all over the place. I walked very slowly and carefully. I must have looked as scared of falling over as I felt. People looked at me oddly in the lift and corridors, and solicitously moved out of the way.

Two hour drive home from London in the rush hour traffic. Only one near miss, when someone almost went into the side of our car on a roundabout. What a day for that to happen! Never mind. Home now. Bed as soon as I got in.

23rd August

Flowers arrived from my sister. I am so thankful. I never used to like cut flowers in the house, preferring to look at them in the garden, but I think I have been converted.

It is very odd lying in bed on my left-hand side, because I can't feel my ear, and it feels like I am lying on something. I have to turn over a sleep on the other side.

24th August

Feeling very sick today. Still taking the paracetamol and Neurofen the nurse gave me.

Lay in bed till lunch, and went back again at teatime.

I am dealing with this convalescence so much better than the last time. I think it is because I am determined not to let it beat me this time. Last time was rather a novel experience, and I was making the most of it because I knew I wasn't really ill. Now I know what the score is, and I know how hard I can push my body. I also know that I can't do anything worse to it than has already been done. I am trying to ignore the facts of what is happening, and carry on as normal. Either I'll sail through, or fall over completely. We will see.

25th August

My mother phoned yesterday, and when I complained about feeling sick, she suggested I stop taking the Paracetamol. It makes her sick, and she thinks it might be doing the same to me. Why couldn't she have told me this two operations ago? I have stopped taking it now, and do feel better.

26th August

Quick visit from my parents today. It really brought home to me the fact that I am still quite ill. I wanted to go out to the local garden centre and to the shops, and I couldn't. I really couldn't. I am still too weak. I am padding round the house as slowly as I like, I forget what the real world is like, and the speed at which it turns. I am in a little world of my own here. A slow little world, that potters along making cups of tea and occasionally weeding a small patch of garden. I don't know how I am going to cope with going back to work. Should I be making plans to strengthen myself up? Should I have a stringent exercise and eating regime, to bring a spring to my step and roses to my cheeks? Or should I be resting quietly and 'getting my strength up' that way? Perhaps some Complan would help? What I do realise is, that I can't take it too quickly. My body will heal at its own rate, and I must allow the inside bits to heal before I push it too far too fast on the long and winding road to recovery. Another cup of tea, vicar?

27th August

Today I played nurse to myself and took some of the steri strips off my neck. I was so worried that it was going to tear the wound open that I picked and pulled very gingerly. I have taken off every other one, not so much because I think they need to stay there, but as a psychological sop to myself, so that I know I won't pop open and start to spill bits of my insides everywhere. I shall take the rest off tomorrow. I have to say that it does look loads better without the covering. How can it heal so quickly? Aren't human bodies wonderful? And I suppose animal bodies are wonderful, too, truth be known.

28th August

Claire came home today. She has been away since I had the operation. I hope she wasn't too upset at seeing me look so grey and puffy still. I think she has got used to me being ill now.

29th August

Went to visit an art exhibition this afternoon. What a mistake. I am still SO WEAK! I thought that a little wander round would be the same as walking round the house. How wrong can you be? I was so exhausted that I had to make use of the carefully placed chairs that were put out for the elderly and the infirm. I felt really silly, but couldn't help myself. I would have fallen over completely if I hadn't stopped to rest.

30th August

Sitting in the shade sipping an ice cold drink with a slice of lemon in it. What could be nicer? Well, being allowed in the sun without fear of being left with a huge red scar would be nicer. Being able to get up and mow the lawn would be nicer. feeling that moving the guinea-pig cage was a possibility would be nicer. Having brown legs to look down at, from having sunbathed earlier in the year would be nicer. Shall I go on?

31st August

I have a great deal of respect for the doctor who did my operation. It has come out more like cosmetic surgery than necessary bludgeoning. Is that too harsh on the previous doctor? Probably. How nasty of me. This last doctor has followed the lines in my neck (how lucky I have so many for him to choose from!) very nicely, and I am hoping the scars will hardly show once they fade, and as my natural lines get deeper.

I have started to have hot flushes at night. I have heard, on the grapevine – or was it the Internet? – that radiation treatment and/or surgery can start off the menopause. I shall have to look it up.

September – a month of misty, mellow fruitfulness. An uncertain calm, followed by a stormy squall.

1st September

Should have gone to a barbeque this afternoon, but was too ill. I was going to go, and just sit quietly in a corner, and then I decided that that was a silly idea, and it would be better not to go at all. If I had gone and decided to come home early, everyone else would have had to, too. Sat in my own garden instead.

Funnily enough I am not worried about dying any more. I seem to have got over that little hurdle.

2nd September

Received this email today:

> *Hello. I am in the UK too. I had a TT, radiotherapy, RAI and also a neck dissection. My ears were numb but the feeling has come back now. I am just numb around my Jaw line and it tingles! I live in London and have pap thyroid cancer, poorly differentiated. I hope you feel better after your latest ops. I have a wonderful surgeon too - hardly a scar shows and they have been in three times! and I also had a tracheotomy for three months and also my vocal chords are paralysed. Oh well.All the best,*
>
> *Merle*

However ill you are, there is always someone worse off.

3rd September

Put a note on a message board on the internet asking if anyone else had found that the treatment sparked off the menopause.

I am calling this year my Annus Horibilis.

4th September

Wasn't it only a few days ago that I was saying how perky I was. Had a down day today. There doesn't seem to be much rhyme or reason for this. Perhaps an outsider would notice a pattern. I think it is because I can't sleep properly. I have bought some herbal tablets to help me sleep.

I am finding it hard to put my earrings in because my left ear lobe is still numb. I usually do it by touch, and can't do that now, so I have to reach round in front of a mirror to see what I am doing. I am rather afraid of jabbing myself with the sharp end, and not realising. Roll on the return of the senses.

5th September

Went to see my lovely consultant again today, and he says he wants to do more radioactive iodine treatment. I think that is OK. It takes a while to sink in. I don't think I am in a position to refuse treatment. He had previously said he would do it in November, but he has now brought it forward to October. I find that worrying. He is going to give me a larger dose this time.

I asked him if I still needed to pay into my pension fund, and he laughed. The real question, obviously, was, 'am I going to die?' He said I should keep paying it. Was this an off-the-cuff reply, and can I take it as a certainty that I am going to last another 20 years? The mortality figures show I have only a 70% chance of lasting that long. That means one out of three will die. What makes him think I won't be one of those?

Once again, I come out of a meeting with him smiling and shaking hands and thanking him, and not really 100% conscious of what I am doing/saying. My mind is still going over and over what he has told me. Why has he brought the date forward? Why is he giving me more, if there is now less cancer in my body since the surgery? Does this mean I am more ill than I realised? Will I die? When will I die? Will this cure me? How long before it comes back again? If it comes back, will the treatment be even worse than this time round? Are you sure I'm not going to die? I don't believe you.

6th September

I tell Claire that I have to have more radiation treatment. She knows this is not good, and that it means I am not cured. We all thought the surgery would be the end of it. She has now started worrying about my survival again.

Ordered my shopping from an online supermarket today. What a good idea. I wish I'd done it before. I even had a money-off coupon, and won't have to pay for delivery. Great. I can sit back and wait for a little man to deliver it. Ah, the life of an autocrat – 'you, boy, bring food!'

7th September

It's now beginning to get chilly, and dark in the evenings. Where has my summer gone? I am going to 'lose' most of this year. It will become 'The Year That Never Was'.

Got a reply to my online queries about the menopause:

> *Hello Sue*
> *I got my periods back. I found after the RAI they were Irregular and missing and then got them back. I was sweating but that is probably the T3 I*

was on and RAI. Now have them every six weeks but my blood tests do not suggest that I am in the menopause. My last period came on time. My endo says it is because of all the stress etc. After all, your hormones take a terrific bashing

Best wishes, Merle

8th September

Walked across the road to get a newspaper from shop opposite my house today. It seemed like such a bit step! I hate being so weak all the time. There is such a lot to do, and it's not getting done.

9th September

Colin and his sister came today to help me do a garden makeover. It's great being ill. I drew out the design on paper, and then stood and watched while they did all the hard work. When everything was ready, I stepped in and did the planting. Oh, this has its good points.

I picked up a magazine today with a feature article on breast cancer fundraising. Three celebrities were featured as supporters of the campaign, but none of them had had breast cancer themselves. It got me thinking, and I came to the conclusion that generally speaking it's not people who have had cancer who campaign most ardently for funds to find a cure. It's people who have lost loved ones to the disease, and are there fore afraid of getting it themselves. They hope that a cure will be found before they get it. People who have cancer fundraise for hospitals and hospices, to maintain equipment and pay nurses, not for a cure.

I always used to be so positive in my thinking, and now the latent cynicism that I suppose lies somewhere in us, all has come out. It is usually suppressed by inbred rules of 'proper' behaviour.

10th September

I wish I'd measured the circumference of my neck before I went in for the surgery in March. It is so much thinner now, especially as the swollen lymph nodes have been removed. I have thought for years that I have a short neck, but I realise now that that isn't the case at all. It was all an optical illusion brought on by the fact that my neck was a lot wider than it should have been.

I have been trying on some of my Jewellery again, which I had got out of the habit of wearing. It looks a bit silly with a big red scar, as if I am highlighting it. I am pleased to be able to wear it again, though. Perhaps I'll even start buying more. What I need is a fancy man who will bring me diamonds.

11th September

I have been trying to do some planning for the future. I am finding it hard, as I don't know when I will be ill again. I have come to believe that I will be ill again; as a recurrence is quite likely once you have had lymph node involvement. The question is- when? The speed that my life is whizzing past at the moment, I am going to be at the end before I know it. What then? What will I think when I look back? Will I think I have played a full and useful part in society? The sensible thing to do, is to plan and get on with it all quickly, but to have a contingency plan pencilled in, just in case. How mature and sensible. How unlikely to happen.

12th September

Today, a switch clicked inside me, and I acknowledged to myself that I have to go into hospital for the radioiodine treatment again, and thought about the full implications. Had a little cry. Thought again about overall thyroid cancer survival rates, and worked out that 70% survival is 2:3.

However many times I do the maths, it still comes out the same. Oh well, can't change it. What I find it hard to get my head around, is the fact that the percentage doesn't change as your treatment progresses. I suppose that you inch towards the survival group instead of the mortality group, though – a bit like a leader board.

13th September

Today I have been feeling little tingly feelings along my jaw line, like tiny sparks of lightening. I think it must be the feeling coming back. I hope so. The feeling still isn't back from my ear, and it still feels odd to sleep on it.

14th September

I have grudgingly put all the little green labels back on the food in my cupboard to show which is allowed on the LID diet, and taped up the list of 'free' foods on the wall. I am much more prepared than I was before, but I am still not keen on doing it. I do feel grateful that we seem to be in a much better position than the Americans. We seem to have loads more healthfood shops, and vegan/vegetarian books to help us. If I was keen, I'd start baking/cooking casseroles for the freezer. I'm not.

15th September

I have been on the Internet today, putting all my books up for sale. I have amassed so many since I have been ill, I don't have anywhere to store them. I suppose they really ought to go down to the charity shop. I am not as selfless as I used to be, and I am going to get something for them if I can. Magazines have gone to the doctors surgery as I finished them, so I give myself a team point for that. Soon have my socially-responsible-citizen badge.

Emailed a friend in Holland, letting her know how it was going, and to get some advice about publishing my LID diet notes. She wrote back:

> *Your life does seem to be full of horrible machines and alphabet soup(PET, CT). Not easy to be sunny when you're living through all that.*
> *Judith*

Well it's nice that she thinks I am sunny. Not sure about living in a land of alphabet soup, though – could get a bit sticky!

16th September

I heard someone talking on the radio this morning, who was comparing the way we live our lives with putting together a DIY shelving unit. He pointed out that almost everyone tries to make the unit without reading the instructions, only resorting the manual when it all goes wrong. He was suggesting that we should all read a 'manual for life', whether it be the teachings of a religious leader or some other work, sooner rather than later. What a waste of time to try to live a useful and sensible life after it has all gone wrong. How much better an idea to read the manual first, and get it right from the beginning. If only it were that simple.

17th September

I'm getting quite lonely now. Very few people come and see me, and I think the people at work have forgotten that I exist. It's interesting to see which people have taken the trouble to stay in touch, and I have to admit that it's not necessarily the people that I thought it would be. When you have a busy life, people that aren't there tend to drift off into the background altogether. I know, I've done it myself.

18th September

I have some good news to report today. I seem to be getting some symptoms of having a period: PMT (rife) and also swelling breasts (slight). The hot flushes haven't abated, but I am trying to put that at the back of my mind (easier said than done at 2am). I sleep with both windows wide open to try and keep cool in the night. Sheesh!

19th September

One of the things that frighten me about the future is the loneliness. I don't mind dying, somehow I've managed to come to terms with that, but I am worried about dying alone. I suppose if (when) I get terminally ill, I'll go into a hospice or home, but I do think about becoming a sad little old lady alone in her own dirty home. Perhaps now is the time to cultivate lots of friends and neighbours? Am I hypocritical enough to make lots of new buddies so that I won't have a funeral with nobody there? I don't think so. Well, I like to think not, anyway…Perhaps when it comes to it, I will. Perhaps when it comes to it, it will be too late.

20th September

Been on the scales again today, and not only am I keeping the weight off, but I have lost another two pounds. Great. If I loose another few ounces, I can say that I am eight stone something. 8st 13lb, but still, it will start with an eight and not a nine. Now that *would* make me happy.

21st September

Oh, the drudgery of being at home all day. At first there was a certain pride in keeping my dear little house nice. Now it just seems boring. It all seems to get dirty/untidy/messy as soon as the work is finished. Will it never end??? It was much better when I was at work all day, and not here to see it.

I have also started to try and cook proper meals instead of ready prepared ones, and that makes more washing-up, too.

22nd September

I have got into the habit of having a bath in the middle of the afternoon. This is when it all seems to get on top of me, and I feel in need of some relaxation therapy. I have started to use a lovely set of aromatherapy candles that I got for Christmas, and have been saving. Why do we do that? Things are given to us to be enjoyed, not put on a shelf. I do get quite a lot of enjoyment out of looking at all my pretty bottles, though, and when they have been used, they'll disappear. I must try and get myself out of the habit soon, because there won't be a bath in the RAI room, and I want to avoid any extra stresses (such as wanting a bath and not being able to have one).

I must also get out of the habit of eating all the time. Being at home, I have started to snack continuously from about 10am through to dinner time. I can report that I haven't put back any of the weight I lost in March/April, when I had my operations, but there's always the possibility. (I must start doing some exercises soon, too)

23rd September

I went up to London today, to see my nice consultant. He had a feel of my neck and is very happy. I think he was only interested in seeing how good his scars look!

He did notice that the right side of my face is quite swollen, and I had to admit that the reason for it is my night-time habit of grinding my teeth. I know I should do something about it, and I did go to the dentist when I had the problem before. He said that it was a habit, and could be broken by wearing a shield at night. Sure enough, a few months after wearing a horrible shield at night, made out of pink plastic the same colour as 1950s NHS glasses, I stopped. I think it was possibly because I hated wearing the shield so much. Anyway, I am hoping that once the stress of having the RAI has gone, the teeth grinding will stop.

The consultant said he took out thirty-four lymph nodes, taking out some either side of those that were obviously infected, but the pathology report has come back saying that only nine contained cancerous cells. Colin was very pleased with this, but I don't consider it a bonus. They've already done the operation, so this new in formation doesn't affect that. And they knew where the cancer was from the scans, so I don't know why it seems like a surprise to anyone. It's probably coming back anyway. I suppose at least I won't be getting a recurrence in the lymph nodes that have now been removed. Now there's a thought. Given that lymph node involvement seems to indicate a higher likelihood of recurrence, and given that one might have had all the lymph nodes removed, does this mean that the cancer will move elsewhere? Hypothetical, I know, because it's very unlikely that anyone will have ALL their lymph nodes removed. I do like to know the answers to questions like these.

He also took blood from me to check if I really am going through the menopause (44, for goodness sake!) or whether it could be something else. I asked him for something to help me sleep between now and the RAI, but he was loathe to prescribe something that is potentially addictive. He thinks I can manage another three weeks on vodka and over-the-counter herbal sleeping pills. Perhaps I should up my dose? Too many, and I'll wake up feeling like a Russian plant. Or perhaps I won't wake up at all.

24th September

What a lot of adverts there are for cancer charities on daytime television. I am always interested to see which adverts come during which programmes, because it gives an insight into the type of person they think will be watching e.g. nappy and face cream adverts during Love Story, Poligrip and Saga during The Bridges of Madison County. Why are they targeting people at home during the day with cancer ads? Do they think that people during the day have more disposable income? I think they'll probably have less, or do they think that these people watch more often, and that they will wear them down? Or do they think that these people have more time to ring up and donate? We'll never know.

I've noticed that the cream prescribed to me by the consultant for my 'menopausal symptoms' is labelled as 'estrogen'. Where is the 'o'? Even the spellchecker wants to put an 'o' in it. I noticed a while ago that the 'a' has gone from mediaeval, and now I see that the 'a' has disappeared from faeces and the 'o' from foetus. Where are these missing letters going? This is all part of a 'dumbing-down' of the English language. I am all for Plain English, in certain places, but I also like correct usage. It's like wearing jeans during the day, but dressing up for important occasions. If language isn't used properly, it will fall into misuse. The language I grew up with as a child will become something like the language of Chaucer – unreadable, and only studied at school by people who have to guess the pronunciation. Oh well, I suppose it's development.

25th September

It's quite chilly today. I think my days of lazing around in the sun are over. It's not going to be so much fun being off work it I have to sit here on my own in the cold each day. I suppose I could always put the heating on, but it seems rather early in the year. I'll go check the weather forecast. It's not as if I can do a lot of exercise to keep myself warm. Sniff.

Claire offered to go on the LID diet with me today. I thought that was really nice of her, and has made me think that perhaps she does has some kind of sympathy for me, in her own teenage angst-ridden way. Or is that just a mother's fondness?

A friend has been trying to get me to apply for a mobility allowance. I have told her that I don't need it, and that I am not ill, but she keeps insisting that I apply, as it takes 3

months to go through the system. I keep repeating that I am not that ill. She says I will need it in the future. I tell her that I am going to get better. She repeats that I will need it later. I repeat that I am trying to keep a positive attitude, and think that I am going to get better. I know she has my best interests at heart, but I ended up in tears. It seems so odd for someone to be suggesting that I am so ill I won't be able to dress myself or walk. I know that she is wrong, and that I will recover this time, but it has given me a 'chilling vision of the future'. One day, I will be in that position.

26th September

I am really beginning to worry about going into hospital again. You'd think that I'dfeel better about it, having been in before, but it makes it worse, somehow. It's the loneliness of it I'm worried about. Well if David Blaine can do it for days underground and weeks in a box, then I'm sure I can manage a few days, too. Perhaps it will be a life-changing experience (another one), and I'll come out knowing the answer to life, the universe, and everything. 42?

27th September

Once again, I have woken up in the middle of the night, having had a nightmare. I shan't take children's nightmares lightly again. I think we, as adults, forget the intensity that wakening to a false reality can have.

I have been waking up the past few nights absolutely sure that I have omitted to do something, and won't be able to go into hospital. It is all very hazy now I am awake, but it seems that my unconscious mind thinks that I am going back for surgery. There is a collection or a delivery that I was meant to do, that has not been done. Yesterday, I woke up calling out. Today I have woken up with a sore throat from sucking my breath in as I wrenched myself back to the real world, sitting bolt upright at the same time. This is what I have been asking the doctor for sleeping tablets to cure. I have made myself a hot milky drink, and will go back to bed in a while, after playing a computer game or two. I can't go straight back, as I am still feeling the effects of the adrenaline in my system. Roll on RAI – once it's over I can sleep again.

28th September

It's a funny thing, but I've noticed that I'm not worried about dying any more. It has been a constant worry to me for so long, I've pushed it to the back of my mind, and now it's odd that it's not there. I am worried about going into hospital, because I wake in the night shouting. Exactly what it is I am worried about, I can't put my finger on. I think I have had enough of it all. Enough of being out of control. I used to be such a 'control freak', needing to know the ins and outs of everything. Now, I am much more likely to let things go. I can see the larger picture, and in the grand scheme of things, our little everyday arguments and niggles don't mean a thing.

29th September

Popped into work this afternoon. Everyone polite and solicitous as usual. It will be hard to go back after wandering around in my nightie all morning, for the past six months. I must give some thought to whether I want to go back to the same job, or whether I want to change it. This might be the ideal opportunity to move across to something else, and the lady who is substituting can continue in my old job. And of course, I can always play it from the 'poor little terminally ill girl' angle. Please be nice to me, I haven't got long to live...

Started the low iodine diet again today. Only one major mishap, when I made my tea with milk first thing in the morning. Well, I was only half awake. I'm fully into it now, and have got my little lists of what to eat and what not to eat stuck up on my cupboard doors. Spent most of today not eating anything at all because I couldn't be bothered to work out what I was and was not allowed. Not having bread or dairy seriously limits the lunch possibilities. I must go and buy a load of salad bits, and have salad every day. How healthy!

30th September

My throat has begun to feel a bit tight, and today my Mother rang and didn't recognise my voice on the phone. I met a lady last week for the first time in two years, and she said my voice had changed, and I took no notice. Can a voice change without you knowing? Do people go on what they see, and discount what their ears hear, so that if they see me, they don't acknowledge changes in the voice they hear? How odd.

I wonder if the operation damaged my vocal chord slightly, and it has taken this long for it to make a difference? Am I slowly losing my voice forever? Or have I just got a cold? Only time will tell.

October – a month of fallen leaves and bonfires, in which our heroine rues her blasé attitude to treatment.

1st October

My ears hurt. It's where I've been grinding my teeth in the night. I wish the RAI was over. I am sinking into a depression that feels a lot like PMT. Nothing is right, I don't feel like doing any housework, and the less I do, the messier it becomes and the more depressed I feel.

I had to turn the heating on today. Not a good sign. No more pottering the in garden and sitting reading as the sun streams in through open windows. I will have to curl up in slippers and a duvet now. And the mercenary side of me says "it's not so good being off sick if it costs you money".

2nd October

I have started to comfort-bake. Some people comfort-eat, I comfort-bake. I have made three cakes recently, and although I can't eat them myself, I have been freezing them. I have also got to be a dab hand at running up home-made bread and lardy cakes. I have a sneaking suspicion that I am turning into Monica Geller, so I am trying to keep the obsessive cleaning under control (and managing extremely effectively, if I say so myself)

Why am I so scared about going into hospital again? I can't see any logical reason why that should be the case.

I know what is going to happen, and it's not that bad. A bit boring, a bit lonely and I will feel rather sick for a week, but nothing so very bad. Each day I get closer to going in, I am getting more and more forgetful, and I keep dropping things. If I had stopped taking the tablets, I would blame it on that, but I haven't, yet. I am so stressed. The other thing that makes me realise I am scared about going in is that I am trying not to think about it, and am putting off organising childcare, and packing my case. The first time, I was all ready and organised days in advance. This time, I keep telling myself I'll do it later. Well, I am glad that I have admitted this to myself now. This is also the first time I have used the word 'scared'. I have always thought of myself as 'worried' before. Denial again, I suppose. So now I know what's wrong with me, there's no reason I can't fix it! Where shall I start?

Sent round an update email to those of my friends who are kind enough to keep asking how I am. I ended:

> *Still smiling here, though.... anyone visiting Carnaby Street can see my paper bowls in Unit 27 Kingly Court. :) TWO exhibitions in October , that I now have to get someone else (Colin) to put up for me, but the see-saw is up that end, even if its down on the health end.*

One of the replies I got was:

> *I keep hearing all those terrible things about you but you seem to be incredibly cheerful. I suppose you always were. I have all my fingers crossed for you.*
>
> *Alan*

This is not the first time someone has said a similar thing to me. Do I appear cheerful all the time? Not a bad thing, I suppose.

3rd October

Drinking tea with hazelnut milk in it. It's OK apart from the smell, and I suppose I'll get used to that. Last time I did this diet it was summer, and I could drink cold drinks. Now it is so cold, I need something hot, so it's either this or black coffee. I'll persevere with the tea.

Stopped taking my triiothyronine tablets today. It's a funny thing, but I found that I was avoiding taking them. It was somehow as if I felt that I needed to make them last, and so should be saving them. I had to make a real effort to take them at the correct time.

Now, of course, I will start feeling ill, as they are my thyroxine substitute tablets. I will start getting slower and slower until I stop, or start taking the tablets again. My whole system will get 'sluggish'.

What a horrible expression. Actually, it probably fits quite well, because with the bloating and the greyness, I'll probably look rather like a slug at the end of it.

Managed to sleep in my normal pre-op sleeping position last night. Heaven.

4th October

Life is going really slowly for a change. Since March, I have felt like life is rushing past me, but now it's suddenly slowed down. It must be something to do with the fact that I am marking time now until I go into hospital again.

My new diet has given me dia...dio... a poorly bottom. I hope it's due to the amount of fruit that I've suddenly started eating, and not the hazelnut milk. I can cut back on the fruit, but please don't ask me to go without my cups of tea!

The more I think about it, the more I realise that I am blocking all thoughts of what has happened to me. I am not a psychiatrist, but I suppose this is being 'in denial'. That is how I can be so cheerful in between times, and how I can smile at people I meet and tell them how great I feel. It's because I have no memory of the nasty bits. I find it hard to remember what it was like in hospital, and especially what it was like when I came home. That is also why my life is going so quickly – I have 'missed out' weeks at a time. This is not good. I must have a think about it, and decide whether I need to do anything about it. Perhaps re –reading this diary will help me. Do you think I'll go mad? Will it come back to haunt me later in life if I don't deal with it now? I don't think I've dealt with any of the traumas in my life. Perhaps they'll all come back to haunt me. Gosh.

5th October

I'm a convert to organic peanut butter. It might look like baby poo, but it tastes lovely. I will keep buying it in future, I think.

Feeling very low today, and had a bit of a cry. The first time in ages. I really don't want to go back into hospital. I have had enough of being ill now. Every time I start to get better, they make me go back in, and I'm fed up with it. I'd just like to be well for a little while in between times, before I have to go through it all again. I haven't been 100% since March, and I am beginning to feel the strain. I am trying hard to look forward to November , when I will be able to go back to work again, but I can't see past the RAI. I hate feeling sick. I would rather be in pain than be nauseous. At least a good clean pain in something you can fight against feeling sick is so debilitating, and yet it's not a 'proper' illness. Not one that makes you feel justified in being off work, or deserving sympathy. Wallow, wallow, wallow.

6th October

I have had hiccups every day for the past three days. Why is that? Is it a little known side-effect of cancer that has been ignored by the medical profession? I should write a medical paper on it, and I could be famous. That'll make up for it.

My diet is going well. Lost two pounds so far. It really makes it easy if you always have the knowledge in the back of your mind that if you cheat, you'll die. Also, a lot of the food is so unappealing that it makes you lose your appetite, anyway. Was rather tempted to cheat and have milk in my tea, but I decided that once I did that, it would make it easier to cheat again, so I resisted. I hope everyone is very proud of me.

Claire asked me this morning why I had been crying in the middle of the night. I couldn't answer. I have been doing it so much lately that I don't even wake up any more.

7th October

I am going to get broadband, I think. It's not a lot more expensive than ordinary Internet access. I wish I'd got it when I first went off sick. It would have saved me loads of time on the Internet. But then again, I didn't know I'd be off for so long. If only we could see into the future, how much easier it would be to plan our lives.

Stayed up until 2am talking to Colin about some things that have been worrying me. About how I've forgotten what it has all been like already. About how I keep using the phrase 'worried' when I really mean 'terrified'. About what the future might hold, and how far ahead I should plan. Assuming I'll last another 20 years, that should just about see my mortgage paid off. What a good job all the paperwork was signed three months before the diagnosis., otherwise it might not have gone through. Where would I be living now if that were the case?

8th October

Watched Holby City today for the first time. Thank goodness I didn't watch it before I had my operations. I wouldn't have been so happy going in, had I known what they were going to do. Seeing it after the event, however, it is quite interesting to see what they did, and how they worked. I feel even more admiration for the staff now.

Getting all the signs of being off my tablets now. Very much like PMT. Keep dropping things. Never mind, all the broken crockery can go as hardcore under the new conservatory.

I am becoming a recluse. I have got so used to not seeing anyone all day, and for most of the evening too, that I rarely go out. Not being able to drive for a substantial part of the last six months hasn't helped, either, because I have got used to popping across to my local shop, and not driving anywhere. At least I'll be in practice for the coming two weeks.

The Internet has been a godsend to me. I have always realised that it is a wonderful invention for people who are housebound for whatever reason. Public perception is that it is useful for families physically separated from others, for example in the outback of Australia, but as soon as I started to use it regularly, I realised it was wonderful for those people separated not by distance, but by illness. Women especially seem to find it useful, for some reason. If you can't get out of the house, you still have access to a world of information.and also a world of other like-minded people. If you are stuck indoors caring for family, young or old, or if you can't go out through physical or mental illness, then you can still interact with other people. I recommend it to everyone! Diatribe ended.

9th October

Got invited out to dinner today. Had to refuse because I am on this silly diet. Have agreed to go for 'cocktails and nibbles'.

Crying again tonight. I don't know why the thought of more treatment worries me so much. You'd think I would be used to it by now. But no. Sobbing again, and not sure why. Perhaps having to go into hospital brings home to me the fact that I am not well still, and that it is a serious

think to have. Also, the fact that I am quite lonely here all day by myself makes me thing that it isn't a good idea to go someplace where I will be even more lonely. Well, if David Blaine can do it, so can I.

I was also crying about the fact that I might not get to do all the things I want to with my life. I have an idea that I'd like to do something great and good, to earn my place in society. We all know that we are going to die at some point, but I don't think we consciously recognise the fact most of the time. That is why having a potentially fatal illness makes you re-evaluate stuff, even if you're not given the screen-writers' favourite 'only six months to live!'

You realise when you are on your way 'down' what a long way there is to go, and what a precarious hold we have on sanity and happiness. When you are depressed, a great dark pit seems to hover beneath you, exerting a gravitational pull of its own. Even when you seem to be as low as its possible to go, there is still further to descend if you don't allow yourself to be pulled out.

10th October

A lot better today. Very busy setting up an exhibition, which knocked me for six, as they say. Had to have a little sleep at teatime. Someone said that I looked 'rather grey'.

By the time I went back for the preview in the evening, I had perked up, and people I met said how good I looked (considering). I think it was largely due to the amount of make-up I'd slapped on! Told some people that I was going to have radioiodine treatment, and would be locked in solitary confinement for a week, and they were amazed.

Avoided the wine, crisps, cheese, canapés and various other assorted nibbles during the evening. What was it I had? Oh yes, sparkling water and orange juice. I'd like to say I was sparkling, too, but I don't think I improved quite that much.

My parents came, and met everyone. When I complained about the amount of work it had been, my father said that the angels in heaven were writing in all down. I jolly well hope so, I get little enough recognition in this world (said the bitter, twisted, depressed psychotic thyca patient)

11th October

Bought a jigsaw puzzle to take into hospital with me. All I need to do is beg, steal or borrow one of those rolling sticky mats for doing it on. Otherwise I'll have to break it all up when I come out. At least if I do that, I can have all the fun of piecing it together all over again. Or would it be so soul destroying I'd end up in a sobbing heap on the floor?

I think when I have finished all this, possibly in the spring, when I have had time to think it all through (and got used to being back at work), I will do a bit of thyroid cancer awareness campaigning. I am not sure I want to collect money, but I would like to raise awareness of the disease, and point people to where they can donate. Hardly anyone has heard of thyroid cancer. Even the cancer help sites have it listed under 'other'. One of the ladies at the hospital says that even some of the GPs she deals with don't really know much about it, and she finds they change people's medication as if they were dealing with a normal hypothyroid condition. Of course, with cancer, this

is completely the wrong thing to do. The medication is the same, but given at a much higher level. I think I mostly want to do it for my own good, so that people know what I am talking about, but it should also help people who might have it and not know, like me.

12th October

Almost there. I have bought cat food, guinea pig food and child food, cleaned the house, organised childcare, washed and ironed everything in the house, filled the freezer, and packed a case of goodies to keep me entertained on the long journey ahead. I think I have covered all bases, but there is bound to be something I have forgotten. At least I feel as if I am winning now, and not standing still, frozen in the path of an oncoming tidal wave.

Very, very tired, today, though. Tired to the point of feeling sick from it. Went to a boot fair this morning, and almost couldn't make it round. Had to come home and rest on the sofa. Can't run up the stairs like I normally do.

13th October

I am now in my little room – a smaller room than that which I had last time. Everything taped over once again. Ready to begin my incarceration. The different staff on duty have had different ideas about the stringency of the regulations necessary, and the nurse has dissuaded me from bringing my jigsaw in with me. Never mind, I have loads of other stuff to do, not least my trusty pen and notebook. I feel like I should have a baseball glove and ball with me.

14th October

Too ill to write.

15th October

Still very ill. Have been more ill than every before in my life. After the dose was administered on Monday, I became sick quite quickly, and have been nauseous every since. Never again will I dismiss sea-sickness as a minor illness. I have been SO SICK. On Tuesday, I was completely prostrate with it, unable to get up, turn over, or even speak with the staff without being sick. They tried three different pills, and an intra-muscular injection before finding a tablet that offered some relief. I spent the day dozing and watching the clock, living quite literally from minute to minute. I was sick five times yesterday, before they found something that could stop it. By that time, I was throwing up frothy yellowish curdled stuff. I was measuring my life, not in coffee spoons, but in ten minute bites. Yes, yes, let me go to Lethe! If I ever have to go again, I will ask if they can fix me up to a drip and sedate me for the first 24 hours. Drastic? You try it.

Still sleeping almost all of the time, and very cold. I still have a vivid impression of yesterday in my mind. I felt like I was lying on a large flat plain of moving mud, a landslip, perhaps, which was gradually moving away from under me. Unable to feel emotion, I don't remember that I cared very much, I have this image in my mind of a vast primeval landscape of brown as far as the eye could see, with the discomfiting peeling-off of layers under me, as the world crumbled.

16th October

Only able to write a little bit yesterday. They have released me today, and I am back home. What a relief. It is so much better to be back in your own home environment. So much more relaxing. And I now have a slave to bring me my every desire. Every desire, that is, except to be free of the sickness (the sickness, the sickness!). That is what will prostrate the nation should the Russians ever launch an nuclear attack – radiation sickness. They will have to wade into Britain through a sea of vomit afoot and a half deep. Nothing will work , and by that stage, no-one will care! It will be the easiest take-over ever.

They gave me a scan before I left. I had to be taken in a wheelchair from the ward up to the nuclear medicine dept, which I at first refused. I then realised that two days without food, or leaving my bed have left me rather weak, and I can't even stand up properly. When I lay down on the scan bed too fast, I felt faint. It showed uptake, though how much, I couldn't tell. A lot in the stomach, not surprisingly. I will speak to the consultant about it later. I do hope he considers it a success. What if it was all for nothing? I suppose it had to be tried.

I am left with a very strong flavour of metal in my mouth. I keep eating Marmite sandwiches and drinking lime squash to try and rid myself of it.

Note: I was very upset to get on the scales when I came home and see that I hadn't lost any weight, even though the last meal to stay in my stomach for any significant length of time was Sunday night. Pah! In future, I shall concentrate on being voluptuous instead of sylph-like.

17th October

Didn't wake up until 10 am this morning. That is after going to bed at 8.30pm last night. I have slept almost continually for the last four days. Apart from dozing almost all day, I have been sleeping 12 hour nights. Today, I am still weak, but went to the little shop. I have been told that the radiation will leave my body much more quickly this time, and I will be free of restrictions on Monday. Yay!

Ate proper dinner today. Curry, to mask the metallic taste. I wonder if it is perceived or real? I wonder how you define the difference? As all senses are merely a reaction of the mind to a stimulus, and can be turned on or off (viz. self-hypnosis), then is a psychosomatic symptom as real as one triggered by an external stimulus? (Discuss, in an essay not longer than 500 words. Do not attempt to write on both sides of the paper at once.) (Can one be sued for too much plagiarism? Can one be sued for not being able to spell plagiarism in the first place?)

18th October

I think this taste left in my mouth has something to do with the salivary glands. I know that the mucous areas of the mouth are the last to clear, and I know that some people get problems with their salivary glands, so that makes sense. I have noticed that the taste is not there in the morning, but is most intense after a meal. I have been 'milking' my salivary glands over the basin in the bathroom to try and clear them. I don't know if this is an approved, or even documented, medical practice – I have may have invented something here - but it does seem to clear them. Perhaps I could earn my place in history as a medical genius?

Started back on my thyroxine-replacement tablets today. I had forgotten that I was off these, and this is another contributory factor to my slowing down so badly. It might also explain why I am so very pale. The consultant says they will take 10 days to kick in, but I am hoping to see an improvement before then.

I seem to be working on a different time-table to normal people, now. I can manage 2-4 hours up and about, but then I am totally worn out, and feeling sick, sometimes to the point of tears. I cannot move my legs, and need to sleep. I then sleep deeply for about 4-6 hours. So deeply, that I don't even change position sometimes. I am then ready for another couple of hours awake. I am hoping that gradually the waking times will increase!

19th October

Sleeping two hours out of every four. Very sick. This is what they call 'hypo-hell' – the time when you are off thyroxine, and become clinically hypothyroid. I am pallid, bloated, and look like a hamster. Back to bed.

20th October

Still look like a hamster who's been stuck underground for too long and fed cream cakes – but at least, today, I care. That's got to be better. I now have to decide if I'm well enough to drive myself to hospital for my scan, or whether I need to ask for a lift. I have a suspicion that it's rather like being drunk, when you don't realise that you are incapable. I shall beg a lift.

Went for my scan. Saw the consultant, and now I feel like a million dollars! He said there was little uptake, and although that might mean that I don't take up the iodine well, it was just as likely to be that there was no thyroid tissue to absorb it. Yay! The CT scan in 3-4 weeks will confirm this. Hooray! Then bi-monthly checks for a while, easing off to annual checks in the future. I suppose celebrations are a bit premature, pending the CT scan results, but I feel so WELL considering how I have felt recently, that I am predisposed to optimism. Yes, yes YES! NO MORE RAI! I cannot describe how I am feeling now. (off to open a bottle of lovely, lovely chardonnay)

21st October

Woken up on a high, still. I hardly got any sleep last night – I think I have already slept my quota for the next two weeks. I have been to the shops and bought lots of nice food. Why wait? I smiled at everybody, and they probably all thought I was mad, but what the heck. I have bought flowers and cakes, and everything is lovely. It's raining, and that's lovely. Even the fact that my toilet roll is so fat and fluffy it doesn't fit in the toilet roll holder properly is lovely. It depends which way you look at things, doesn't it? I can quite see why people go away on holiday or have a family party to celebrate when they get the final all-clear after a major illness.

In fact, I have a sneaking suspicion that the consultant knows more than he is telling me, because he didn't show me the results of the scan, like he usually does. I have a feeling he has spotted something, and is waiting confirmation from the next scan. But even that isn't going to dampen my spirits today. Today is for me. I am tempted to scrub my little house from top to bottom and get it all sparkling again, but I know I'm still not back to full health yet. I shall take the opportunity to sit on the sofa, watch a movie, and nibble yummy chocolates. Big smile!

22nd October

Coming down a bit today. Still pretty 'hiked', as they say. Exactly who says that, I'm not sure, but I am sure somebody does, because I don't think I have made it up. Still got the metallic taste in my mouth, and diarrhoea in the mornings, but apart from that, things are looking up. This is certainly the first time since May that I have been able to see and end to this.

Rang round a few people yesterday, and told them that I think it's all over bar the shouting. Perhaps I have been a bit premature, but everyone was very happy for me. I have ten days before going back to work now, in which to spring clean my house (while at the same time, not over-doing it), and completely re-evaluate my life. Should be a doddle. I think I'll have a cup of tea and a sit-down first... wonder what's on TV at this time in the morning?

23rd October

Ha! Exhausted myself yesterday, as everyone warned. Rushed around trying to do six months worth of housework etc in one day, and am completely shattered now. I also spent some time phoning lots of people to tell them how well I am, and spent a good half an hour on the phone to each of them. Hence, a little job that should have taken minutes stretched to many hours.

Today, I must take it easy. I still have mild diarrhoea, and now I have started menstruating as well. Curiouser and curiouser. I shall have to sit quietly and drink milk stout. At long last, I feel like I need pampering. Up until now, I have felt like I wanted to fight it, and to get up and do stuff. Now it's all over, bar the fat lady singing (hopefully), I can relax and allow myself to be ill. Sadly, I only have one week left before I have to go back to work. But that's good, because then I can be a normal person again.

24th October

Talked to Helen again today and she told me it was three years before she got her taste back after having radioiodine treatment! I am hoping mine will be back long before then. I have already lost the metallic taste, and moved on to having no taste at all – what an improvement! It's funny to find out which food has a very narrow taste band. Things like chocolate, for example, just taste greasy. I now only eat really strong things like Marmite and curry (but not together).

We also talked about suitable replies to the inevitable, recurring question "how are you feeling?" The stock answer is a non-committal "I'm OK" or "fine" or "Much better, thank you", but of course it is all relative. Do they mean "How are you, compared to when you were in full health?" or do they mean "How are you, compared to yesterday?" The answers we give are never specific either. We usually unconsciously answer the latter question, with a short, stock answer covering everything from "At least the medication isn't making me throw up any more" to "Well, I was able to drink a cup of tea on my own today". People don't really want to know the details, and quite honestly, we don't want to tell them.

25th October

Spoke to someone today about my hospital stay, and they were horrified to hear that I had been in solitary confinement for four days. I hadn't really thought about it before, being quite an independent person. Having been away from work for so long, too, I have got (or gotten, as the Americans say) used to being alone for long periods of time. I suppose some people are always surrounded by bustle and noise, especially if they come from a large family. I identify more with little old ladies now. I am used to being lonely 70% of the time.

26th October

I have lost a stone since all this began. This is the lightest I've been for ten or fifteen years. I won't say the thinnest, because I am still quite flabby, but a low weight is good. Good for the self-esteem. Thing is, none of my clothes fit now, and I'm not one for rushing out and buying loads of stuff. Would that I were! If I was that way inclined, I could have wardrobes of stuff by now – goodness knows I've had enough reasons to treat myself over the last few months.

Perhaps I could buy a few well-chosen classics. That'll be the day. Perhaps a few agonised-over but badly-chosen final-ditch attempts to go home with at least *something* in the shopping basket even if it doesn't match anything else in the wardrobe. I'll have to get something to wear to work, all my purchases recently have been casual trousers and t-shirts. Great for lounging round the house feeling sorry for myself, but not terribly professional-looking.

27th October

I am now experiencing the psychological effect of knowing its over – and I am feeling good! It's amazing what a lift it's given me. I feel so very different. Everything seems much brighter and better. The future looks rosier, and I am much more optimistic about everything. Wonderful.

Took down an art exhibition today, which I helped to put up two weeks ago when I was off my thyroxine tablets. What a difference! I lifted the same things, but with such ease! I was really surprised at the difference I felt. Although I knew I was tired in the few days before my RAI, I hadn't quite realised what a huge difference it had made.

28th October

Finally, I have realised what's wrong with my taste buds. It's the sweet things that I can't taste. I tested this by eating spoonfuls of stuff from my kitchen cupboard. I even ended up chewing a sugar cube! Nothing! Very very odd sensation. It's a revelation to find out what things actually taste like when you take out the sugar. Marmalade for example – yuk!

I have been wondering whether I should write out a list of things I want to do with my life. What is it they say? If you don't have a dream, how are you going to have a dream come true? If you don't have a goal, how are you going to know you've got there? I think it's more to the point that if you don't have a goal, you stop pushing. You drift. You float. And then you find it's too late. Better get that list started....

29th October

I lay in bed for a long while this morning, thinking how nice and warm it was inside, and how chilly it was outside. I planned my day, decided which jobs to do, thought about the coming week, and I struck me that everything is suddenly back to normal. I haven't been back to work, and I know things will have changed there, but apart from that, nothing seems to have changed. I had somehow thought that this would have been a life-changing experience, and my whole view of the world would have changed. No such luck. It's back to the same old routine day in and day out. The house still needs cleaning, the washing needs doing, and the I must get round to cleaning out the guinea pigs before they pack their little bags and move out altogether. Perhaps one day I'll look back, and see that there were imperceptibly small changes in my thinking that have ultimately shaped my future. Or perhaps I'll look back and think 'what a waste of half a year'.

30th October

I think I am beginning to get dehydrated because I don't like the taste of any drinks. Water tastes especially bad. I am finding that I am thirsty all the time, but don't fancy anything to drink because it all tastes so bad. I must find something like fruit juice or squash that I can add to drinks to make them nicer. At least I'm getting thin because anything sweet tastes like lard.

I had a moment of moral crisis today. I was writing a new CV for my papermaking work, and was wondering whether to make a big 'thing' of having cancer. I'm sure it would help sell stuff – people like to patronise sick people. But would I feel happy playing on my illness like that? Just to sell more work? Other people do. I think perhaps I won't.

31st October

Nothing at all interesting happened today. I suppose we all have days like that. I feel like I am almost a normal person again. Just someone who has 'lost' seven months of their life.

November – a month of fireworks and festivals, in which the finishing tape seems finally to be within reach.

1st November

Not looking forward to going back to work on Monday. I've been off for seven months now. I find it hard to believe it's been that long. I have missed great chunks of time by being ill, I suppose. It's odd in the morning to wake up and feel the chill in the air instead of the warm summer sunshine I've been used to. How odd to have missed almost a year of my life. The times when I wasn't ill, I didn't care enough to think about the seasons, or the passing time, or whether I should be doing something more worthwhile than watching television or reading. Oh well, back to reality.

2nd November

Frantic rush today to get everything ready for tomorrow. The lymph-node-removal scars are hardly visible now, but the thyroidectomy scan still looks quite red and is very noticeable. I am going to have to be ready for people to examine me. I don't mind if they ask, I don't like it very much if they keep sneaking looks and not saying anything. Then you don't know if they are thinking that you look offensive or whether they are just interested. I think everyone is interested in other people's illnesses. People like to think that they would cope better.

3rd November

First day back at work. It is now 7.30pm and I am ready for bed! I think I'll go and have a soak in the bath. One thing that I have started to do since being ill, is to have (take?) aromatherapy baths. I initially did it because I was feeling sorry for myself, and felt that I needed a treat, but then I realised that the candles and the smells do relax you enormously well. I'd like to make some of my own recipe herbal bath bags from plants I grow in my garden. MMmmmm.

4th November

I am SO TIRED! I feel almost as bad as I did after the operations. I have arranged to go into work mornings only for the next week or so, to ease myself in gently. It has made me think about all the things that have happened to me over the last few months, and although my mind is ready (more than ready) to go back to work, my body is not. What is it they say? The mind is willing, but the flesh is weak. My poor old flesh has been cut and sewn, pricked, bled and irradiated so much it has given up altogether, I think. Up the hill to Bedfordshire.

5th November

Bob and Julia's cat has got cancer. They have done what they can for it, and have now decided that it is kinder to have it put down. I am hoping that I will get af forded that consideration when it is my time to go. I have a horrid feeling that it won't be like that. I have heard horrible stories of people being left to starve to death. I must look it up somewhere. Where? I suppose pro-euthanasia groups will have all the goriest details, in an effort to recruit new members. The pro-life sites will have all the arguments for. The truth must lie somewhere in between. I don't think people normally start to consider issues like this until they face death.

Have I faced death? I THOUGHT I was facing death. Does that count? Is a psychological certainty the same as reality? If you believe it, does it make it real? I think it this case, it does. It was real to me. I believed it, and my consciousness has altered as a consequence of that. My life will never be the same. I have done all my thinking about death and dying, and don't need to be afraid of facing it now. That means I have made a step forward. I think there are stages one must go through in life, and acknowledging one's own mortality must be one of them. It's not so bad.

6th November

I spoke at length today to a lady who has had breast cancer, and is still recovering. She sang the praises of the support group she belongs to. I still feel a bit offended that I wasn't offered any support or counselling. Why is that? Did the consultant think I was brave and strong and didn't need any? Wasn't my cancer bad enough? Or did I slip through the net? I suppose I can be proud of the fact that I have come through it on my own. Given the choice, I think I would have tried it that way anyway, being an independent soul. It's always nice to be asked, to the party, even if you don't want to go.

7th November

Someone today asked me about my next scan, and whether I was hopeful about the results. I have been hopeful about the results every step of the way. Perhaps it is that which has kept me going. Naïve? Possibly, but I am sure that my optimistic outlook has helped me not only mentally, but physically, too. It made for rather a rocky ride, going from an emotional high to a depressive low, but at least I had the high times in between. It would have been a long and hard road to travel without those sparkly bits.

8th November

I have got into the habit of taking my thyroxine every morning. I have only ever forgotten to take it on a day when I was at home. I don't know how I would cope if I forgot it, and wasn't able to take it until I got home from work. I think I might panic. I am very conscious that these tablets are suppressing thyroid cell activity, and thereby preventing the growth of any remaining cancer. I suppose this will get easier as the years go by.

9th November

I still come home from work feeling completely washed out. It doesn't seem possible that it was less than a month ago that I went into hospital for the RAI. No wonder I'm not yet feeling 100%.

10th November

I had to come out of a meeting at work today. I got an email before work telling me that Kathy's cancer has come back. I read it quickly, and rushed out of the house without further thought. It must have shown in my face that something was on my mind, because Lesley asked me if I was OK. I burst into tears! We went into the ladies, and I howled. I don't know why I was so upset. Kathy is going for more radioiodine treatment, and will doubtless be OK. Was it the thought that thyroid cancer does come back? Had I been thinking that one clear scan meant it was gone forever? Something in my subconscious mind has made a mistake, and this seems to have put it right. Luckily the meeting was over by the time I'd calmed down, and I didn't have to go back in with a blotchy red face and swollen eyes.

11th November

Getting into the swing of things now. Life is getting back to normal, and I have nothing to do now but wait. Wait for the scan at the end of the month, wait for the results, and then wait each year for more tests to see if it has come back. If it does, this whole episode will start over again.

However, I am NOT waiting to die. Seven months ago, the ground opened up, and I fell into a deep chasm of darkness and fear, from which I thought I would never emerge. I felt like having cancer meant that I would feel like that forever, until I died a horrible death. I now see that there is hope. There is always hope. A prognosis is by its very nature vague, and no-one can ever, ever give you a definite date by which you will be dead.

The way forward is to live with it as a minor inconvenience, interrupting your life, but not changing its ultimate course. DO NOT accept that it will beat you. DO NOT accept that it will stop you doing what you want to.

I know that I can never be free of thyroid cancer, but this 'wake up call' has made me even more determined to make my life count. Another cliché proving to be a valuable insight into life as we know it! I think this Journey has been worth while after all.

(Reading back over that, I feel like I deserve some applause – please clap now)

More tales of November – things start to go awry

25th November

I am so scared. I had a CT scan yesterday. They confirmed that I'd had one before, and then hardly said a word more to me. When I came out, I felt fine, and drove off - five minutes later, I pulled back into the hospital car park, and went back in. The place where they had inserted the canella in my arm to give me the contrast dye had started to bleed, and my jumper sleeve was soaked. Soon fixed with a bit of clean cotton wool.

This is not the reason I am scared.

I have an appointment next week to see the consultant and hear the results of this test, and now it is getting close, I am losing my cool. Four times I have been in this position, and four times I have been told I need to be admitted to hospital for more treatment. Do I go on past experience, and accept that it will happen again, or do I claim that the law of averages dictates a change? If there is still cancer in my neck, I think I will need external beam radiation. Sore neck, burnt throat, living on Complan and soup. I am depressed, I cry a lot, and I have started to research survival statistics again. At least I am looking up survival figures, and not mortality figures. A small point, but significant. Methinks we have been here before.

PS Found out that the bone scan I had in July cost £120, and the 'ordinary' sestimibi scans costs £85. Thank goodness we have the NHS to pay for it all.

26th November

Didn't sleep very well last night. Things are beginning to get to me. I feel silly, because I have nothing definite to be scared of. Yet. The scariest thing is the unknown.

27th November

Off work today. I am getting so stressed about my appointment with the Nuclear Medicine consultant, that I can't think straight. I am making mistakes all the time, and so I came home early yesterday. I have to go in next week, but I'll stay off tomorrow.

28th November

My days are slipping. I can't sleep at night, so I lay in bed in the mornings. Not good. Must get out of this habit. I don't want to do anything any more. Everyone is getting ready for Christmas, and trees and lights are appearing everywhere. I can't get excited about it. Maybe after I have seen the consultant, and know where I stand.

29th November

Spent the morning in bed. Played in the garden this afternoon, planting some fruit trees that arrived in the post. This has given me some sense of 'grounding'. I love my garden, and I especially love the spring when the new shoots appear. Planting things has given me back a sense of the future. How philosophical. It sounds foolish to write it down, but we all need markers to chart our lives. Some people follow the passing of the sporting seasons, or the changing range of foods in our shops. I watch my garden growing and changing each year. A little miracle that I help to happen.

30th November

Went to a Christmas craft fair today, and bought some things for Christmas. I am still feeling rather light-headed, and as if I am from a different planet, but I do see that things need to be done, whether I am ill or not. I shall still be here at Christmas, and if there's not turkey, it will be my fault!

December – a month of carols and rejoicing, and a time to come to terms with the future.

1st December

I haven't been this tired for ages. I feel as if someone has hit me across the eyes with a plank of wood. I keep yawning and almost falling asleep in front of the telly. However early I go to bed, I still wake up about an hour afterwards, and then again in the middle of the night. Perhaps I'll try some herbal sleeping tablets.

2nd December

Well, not sleeping might not be doing much for my appearance, but I'm getting loads of stuff done about the house! It's all sparkly clean due to midnight dusting etc!

3rd December

Beginning to get really scared now about the appointment with the consultant. Luckily, he is very nice, and I trust him. It must be awful to be allocated to a doctor you don't get on with, and don't trust.

I think one of the worst things about cancer is the damage to the cerebral rather than the physical part of you. So far, the treatment has been uncomfortable, but I have not had any pain from the cancer itself. I have suffered mentally, though, from the moment I was diagnosed. Sometimes to the point of near hysteria. It has only pushed to the surface once or twice, but at those times, I have felt complete panic, losing my sense of sight and hearing, and getting lost in my own decreasing circle of reality. I have been with Colin at these times, and I believe that this was a deliberate (if subconscious) decision on my part. One keeps control as long as possible, but if the sluices are not cleared regularly, the dam can break. Luckily, I am still strong enough to shore up the entrances, and return to normality. One thing I am frightened of is 'losing it' forever, and ending up a gibbering, slobbering idiot incarcerated in a Victorian bedlam. I am conscious that this eventuality is never far away. It lurks like a hovering dark shape, just behind my shoulder, out of sight, but nodding to itself. One day it's time will come.

4th December

Slept all through last night – hooray! Perhaps the outpourings of yesterday had a cathartic effect? Whatever the reason, I am grateful.

My friend's daughter has a job calibrating the scanning equipment at the hospital. I wonder if she realises how very important her job is? It could mean the difference between life and death if the machine doesn't pick up something when it should. I wonder how many of us really appreciate the value of the work we do? Repetition of a task, especially over years, often leads to a cavalier attitude. (Perhaps you should write that one down)

5th December

I have been working so hard this week that they days have gone really fast. Arts workshops every day have been really physically tiring, which has helped me to sleep again.

6th December

People have been wishing me 'good luck' at my appointment with the consultant. Bad wording. He is going to tell me what I have or haven't got. Luck doesn't come into it.

7th December

I seem to have started a daily diary entry again. Is this because I have no friends? I think it is because there are very few people who really understand what I am going through. I worry that the people I see on a day-to-day basis will get fed up with my moaning. People do ask me if I am all right, and I always say yes. I think it is obvious I have things on my mind, but there's no point telling anyone, as there are no answers. I will have to wait.

8th December

Ha ha ha ha ha ha ha. Still got it. One little piece of tumour is still nestling under my left collarbone. Seeing as radioiodine doesn't seem to work on me, that means more surgery. I am stunned, and feel like I am walking around in a dream. I feel more shocked than I did after the initial diagnosis.

I wonder why? I feel like I am shaking, and it is odd to look down at my hands and see that they
look steady. The shaking is all on the inside. I haven't slept properly for a week now.

If they want to cut it out from behind my collar bone, they might have to break the bone to get at it. How do I feel about that? Nothing. I feel don't feel anything.

The consultant also reminded me of the danger to my vocal chords. Apparently, we all have two, and only need one to be able to speak normally. They cannot tell at the moment how many of mine are fully functioning, so someone needs to look down my throat to find out. He explained that if one vocal chord was already damaged, they would have to be extra careful of the second. My reply to this was that it didn't matter about saving my voice. If it came to a choice between losing my voice and having cancer, I know the answer straight away! I'd much rather they cut a large margin around the tumour and sacrificed my voice than have to have repeated recurrence and surgery.

I have a friend who has been treated for breast cancer this year. After months of various treatments, she confided that she would opt for a full mastectomy if she was given the choice again. When we are first faced with surgery, we want the doctor to cut out as little as possible, and allow us to remain whole. Afterwards, when there is the possibility that the cancer may return, we change our minds. How cowardly we are when it comes to it. How much we want to live. The initial request to cut as little as possible is made when we are still in a state of semi-denial. We understand the diagnosis, but have not fully come to terms with all that it means. Once we see the sand in the egg-timer running downwards, we soon change our minds. Cut off my ears, my hand, my legs, but let me live.

9th December

Watched a weepie film today in which loads of people died. I don't know why I didn't switch it off. I should have known it would upset me. I do so hope that I will go quickly when I die. That is the 'bottom line' to it all. The dying isn't frightening; it's the pain beforehand that is. If I knew I could die instantly, there would be nothing to fear.

10th December

Had a special tomographic scan today. Seemed much like the others to me – injection in the arm, wait 30 mins, then lie on a narrow bed under a dishwasher. Only difference this time was that they did a side-to-side pass as well as a top-to-bottom one. I looked at the computer screen showing the results, and there seems to be quiet a large bit of tumour left.

I don't mind so much if they missed a bit. Human error, I can forgive. What is frightening is that it might have grown since my surgery in August. Surely the surgeon can't have missed such a large lump. He seemed quite positive that he'd cut it all out.

They have put together a multi-disciplinary team (MDT) to discuss me, and I'll have an appointment next week to hear the results. I don't mind being an 'interesting case' if this mean something out of the ordinary. I don't want to be an 'interesting case' if it is another way of saying 'wildly out of control'.

11th December

Nice consultant phoned me at home. I am booked into St Thomas' Hospital in London on 13th January "if that's all right with me". Well, of course it's all right with me! Nothing is as important as getting this sorted out, and anything else I had booked would have to be cancelled. I suppose he had to ask...

He doesn't seem to think the tumour has grown since the last surgery. The surgeon has admitted that, for whatever reason, he may have missed a bit. I will ask him more about that later. I don't want to think that they are lying to me. Are they allowed to? I have a suspicion that they don't want to tell me the worst, to 'keep my spirits up'. The best was to keep my spirits up is to treat me like an intelligent and valued member of the community, so that I think there is a reason to go on living, not to treat me like an idiot, so I feel worthless.

Once again, I avoided asking him about a long term prognosis.

12th December

Someone asked me today whether I had received any counselling. I told her I hadn't and made light of it, but I am now beginning to feel like I need some. I am not feeling suicidal, but I am edging towards fatalism (I think that is the right term). I feel like nothing I do will ultimately make an impact on the world, so it's not worth doing anything at all. Who will miss me when I am gone? If I didn't do things, wouldn't someone else pick up the baton? It has been proved over and over again this year that I am not indispensable. The things I do will continue to be done. The people I see continue to live their lives without me. I am fighting it, but I feel less and less inclined to do things as the days go by. I have even stopped putting cans and bottles out for recycling, which has for a long time been one of my pet projects. Oh well, I suppose I'll come out of it. And if I don't, then I don't suppose that will really matter, either.

13th December

I told someone today about having to go back into hospital, and she was very sympathetic. When I joked that at least they could save on the anaesthetic because my neck was still numb from last time, she didn't take it so well. I don't think she knew how to respond. I am meant to be a sobbing wreck, or a stiff-upper-lipped stoic. I don't think I am expected to be my normal self. I know I have bouts of crying and depression (who wouldn't?), but in between, I have to carry on as normal, and it's normal for me to crack Jokes. People will just have to live with it (however bad they are).

14th December

People keep asking me if they can visit me in hospital. I know they are being kind, and I feel bad saying no. I'd rather they came and visited while I am recuperating, and getting bored. I suppose that's not so exciting for them, though.

15th December

Someone else's mother has died. It happens all the time. What will become of Claire if I die? Where will she live? Who will look after her? Should I start to write little letters to her for when she is older? Make a memories box? Perhaps I'll wait.

16th December

I have started buying books written by people who have cancer, and about coping with cancer. This is the first time I have felt the need to do this. Whether or not I read them is a different matter. I have stacked them neatly next to my bed. When I finish my current (detective) book, I will look at them again, and decide.

I don't know if it counts as giving up, this looking for help and inspiration. I am desperately afraid to let go. One thing that has sprung out of all the emails people have sent me, and comments they have made, is how well they think I am coping. This is because I feel like I am standing on the edge of a precipice, and that if I look down, I will fall. Once or twice, I have glanced down, and felt the terror closing in around me. Luckily, a few minutes of hysterical sobbing has always brought me back to reality. Or at least, to the reality I want to see. Is this healthy? Should I face up to it? Will this make it less frightening? Or will the full horror of it all be too much for me? At this moment, I still don't exactly know what the 'full' horror is, even.

17th December

I know have a week off before Christmas. I can't muster any enthusiasm for it this year. I don't know if it's because I have other things on my mind, or if it's because I am getting old. Too many Christmases each the same for any of them to be special. I should think myself lucky that the consultant(s) didn't think that my cancer was the fast-growing type, and use that as an excuse to have a really huge, expensive Christmas-time. The sensible me thinks that I'd regret it afterwards. I still can't help feeling that there has been a mistake, and that I'm not seriously ill after all. It's like waking up in the middle of the night, still half-asleep, and not really knowing the difference between the dream-world and reality. Sometimes I think it would be just as easy to wake up in the wrong one. Perhaps we do live in the dream land?

18th December

Rang the hospital today to confirm my appointment. They are taking me in on Tuesday, but not operating until Wednesday. I might book in one of my many visitors to the Tuesday night to keep me company.

19th December

I got a Christmas card today from an old college friend. We exchanged email addresses, and caught up with the news. She has had so much illness in the last ten years, that it's amazing she is still going strong, and happy with her life. It made me feel quite embarrassed to be worried about one little operation. It just goes to show: there's always someone worse off than yourself (again).

20th December

I have realised that I have slipped into drinking a lot more than I ever used to. I rarely used to drink at all, and now I have something every night. I have been drinking alcopops, but have now invested in a bottle of vodka and some mixers instead – much more economical. And where did I put that meths ...?

21st December

Started reading John Diamond's book today, and although I have only ready the introduction, I think that buying it is one of the best things I have ever done. It is so nice to read someone else's experiences. I think that a book can be more honest than a face-to-face encounter. Even when talking to someone who has had the same experience as you, there is always the unspoken obligation to remain positive, and give encouragement. So who can you turn to? Just Kitty. It doesn't matter that there is no reply, because most questions cannot be answered anyway, and many are simple rhetorical.

22nd December

I am beginning to get back some sense of my responsibility to society. This has manifested itself in a regeneration of my almost fetishist approach to recycling. I am Recycling Woman. Cardboard, glass, cans, paper, compostable scraps, milk bottle tops, stamps – you name it, I collect it and recycle it. Since being a bit depressed this autumn, that had gone by the wayside, but I am now able to report to you that recycling is alive and well in the wilds of Eastern Kent. This must be good. It means my subconscious has once again recognised that it might live long enough to make an impact on the world. I don't think I will live long enough to reap the benefits of my recycling – that won't be felt until hundreds of years in the future – but I will live long enough to regret not have done it. Hurrah for me – back in the land of the living.

23rd December

I continue to read John Diamond's book '*C, because cowards get cancer too…*' So much of it reflects the thoughts that I have put down here, it is uncanny.

Hardly slept a wink last night. Don't know if it's because I'm excited about Christmas or worried about the operation. I have a sneaking feeling it's the operation.

24th December

Well, so much for my idea of improving my diet to help my body fight the remaining cancer. I have stuffed myself with every imaginable goody today. No Christmas dinner, which at least counts as 'real food', to fill me up, just sweet and biscuits. And I don't care! Another two days, and I'll be good…

25th December

I have given up reading John Diamond's book. He died, didn't he?

26th December

I'm fed up with Christmas now. Too much heavy food, and too much TV. I have gone back to doing much the same as I usually do on a day off.

27th December

Visit to parents today. They are more ill than I am, with colds and sore throats. It's nice that I can be sympathetic to someone else for a change.

28th December

Well, Christmas is over, and there is nothing now between me, and the operation on January 13th. That is rather scary. I was pushing it out of my mind before, in true Scarlett O'Hara fashion, telling myself that I'd think about it later. Now it is the next thing on my to-do list.

29th December

Got up late today, and at 9.10am - found a letter on my doorstep telling me I had a hospital appointment at 9am! Dated and sent 24th December, I don't know how they thought it was going to get here on time. Why not use the telephone?

Anyway, I went this afternoon to see the Ear, Nose and Throat specialist and he gave me a vocal chord check-up. He wrapped tissue around my tongue, tugged on it, and then expected me to be able to recite vowels! I was only with him a few minutes, and he says I am fine. So that's a relief.

30th December

I have had another incisive insight into the nature of human relationships. I have realised that when people ask someone how they are, they are only enquiring about that person's physical state. Very rarely do people ask about how you are feeling. The people that do so get a reputation for being a Good Samaritan, or a fairy godmother.

Is this because we are only able to sympathise with physical pain? Or is it because physical symptoms have their limitations, and psychological pain does not? Is it because we are afraid of opening the floodgate to something we cannot cope with? I suppose that asking about a person's mental well-being can be tantamount to poking a stick into a physical injury. You don't hurt someone by asking about his or her body, but you can hurt them by reminding them of things they were trying to forget. You can see someone struggling to climb a step, and can usually tell if they want help or not. In the absence of visual clues to anyone's state of mind, we tend to avoid mentioning it.

Another reason I think people ignore mental issues is because we all have a mental image of the stereotypical hypochondriac who spends twenty minutes telling you how they are, when two would have done. If someone starts to bleed, you call professional help. If someone starts to cry, you have to deal with it yourself.

January – a month of snowballs and resolutions, in which the knife is once more plunged into the neck of the victim

1st January

New month, new resolutions. I have been looking at what I want to achieve in the coming year, and find that I am limited by the uncertainty of any future treatment. I don't mind booking things that I can back out of, but I don't want to a) let anyone down or b) lose money. Either of these could happen if I agree to stretch myself too far.

This puts me in a dilemma. On the one hand, I have the above to consider, and yet on the other hand, I want to set myself goals. I need to know that I am achieving something in this world, and that it is worth carrying on. If I drop all my previous activities, I know I will sink into depression. Not good for everyday health, and not good for cancer-fighting. Apparently a fit and active mind is as important as a fit and active body infighting the disease.

Let's hope 2004 is better than 2003.

2nd January

I wonder what Samuel Pepys wrote about on the days when nothing happened? I have to admit to not having read his diaries, or even extracts from them, but I gather they are a full and detailed account of his every action. Looking back on my diary, I see that there are chunks of my life left out. Well, we've had Diary of a Breast, now we have Diary of a Thyroid. Or rather Diary of a Space Where a Thyroid Should Have Been.

3rd January

I have realised that I keep using the word 'just'. This is part of my instinct to minimise the severity of the situation. I have removed most traces.

4th January

My daughter asked me to paint her bedroom today. It only took me a few hours, and it gave me such a boost. Not because I've done a particularly good job, but because I was physically able to do it. Last time I tried to do any decorating was in April, after my first operation, before I was a medical expert, and knew all about convalescence and recuperation etc. Back then, I had needed a rest after every couple of brush-strokes. This time, I kept painting until it was done! Hooray for me!

5th January

I am still taking time to research thyroid cancer on the Internet. I am not sure exactly what I think I will find out that is news to me. However, I did find out today that the life-expectancy of someone with anaplastic thyroid cancer (i.e. the fast-growing, resistant to radioiodine kind) is about six months.

So I can't have that, or they would have told me. Wouldn't they?

6th January

I cried in the supermarket this morning. I think it must be the stress of waiting for the operation getting to me. Overall, I am very pleased with myself, and the way I have been coping with having cancer. When I have one of these silly breakdowns, it always surprises me. The catalyst this time was a visit to the toilet (please skip forward if this subject offends you).

Ten years ago, I moved house, and my bowel habits changed. I knew that ideally, I should have told my doctor, but it seemed that it was most likely to be a response to the change in water, stress of the move, etc. The change was merely that I needed to empty my bowels first thing every morning. Since the removal of my cancer, this has stopped, so I realise now that it was my body trying to flush out the infection.

This morning, I suddenly felt that I had to 'go'. No problem. Visited the ladies, and everything seemed fine. What I hadn't bargained for, was the intense emotional response I had. I realised I was scared silly. My unconscious mind had decided it was an indication that the cancer was taking over again. Pushing it to the back of my mind worked for a while, but when I started to explain to Colin why I seemed pre-occupied, I started to cry. I felt much better after I had explained it to him. Bringing it out into the open showed the true size of the problem (in this case minimal) instead of keeping it lurking, un-named in the shadows of my mind. Hopefully, once the Christmas bingeing is over, my lavatorial habits will return to their normal erratic routine.

7th January

Heard a wood pigeon this morning. It was early, and I lay in the half-darkness, drifting through that cloudy place between waking and sleeping, with just the cooing to call me back to the real world. There were pigeons outside my window when I was a child, and I love the sound of their calling. Snuggled in the warmth of my duvet, it relaxed me completely before having to wake up and face the day.

8th January

Had a heated discussion with Colin today. We were talking about the way my relatives had made light of my illness when we met over the holidays.

"I'm sure you'll be fine" they all said. How do they know? I understand that they mean they HOPE I will be fine, but it did make me feel that they were telling me how to feel, and that I was wrong to worry about it. Somehow, it was as if they were taking something away from me. It's not that I am basking in the attention it brings, but it doesn't help to have your fears belittled. With everything else I have to worry about, I don't need to feel that I am over-exaggerating things. I need people to endorse my right to be frightened.

Once again, I came up against the Catch 22 situation of needing Colin's support, and finding that he needed mine. I can only find comfort if I first get him to acknowledge that my fears are legitimate, and this means that he has to face facts that he would rather push to the back of his mind. The way this works, is that I deal with it myself for as long as I can, and then have a wild crying session. Not ideal, but at least we are both still sane.

9th January

People at work have been wishing me luck for next week, and I've been hugged and kissed more than ever before. I still can't quite believe it's happening. I haven't arranged anything for while I am in hospital.

The first time round, I was Mrs Efficiency. I arranged child-care, stocked the freeze, packed, stopped the milk etc, all in plenty of time. Second time, I still hadn't unpacked from the first visit. Third time, I at least worked out what I was going to take in with me, so that I didn't wear it, even if I didn't pack early. I like to do it well in advance, so I have time to remember all the bits and pieces I normally forget.I am putting it off until the very last minute this time.

10th January

Bought a magazine today to take into hospital with me. I am still running after my own tail, trying to do the next four week's housework in ten days. Do I have to stock the freezer for every single day? Surely Claire can go to the shop opposite and buy her own dinner some days? Does it make me a 'bad mummy' to even think that?

Someone has given me 'Birdsong' to read while I am convalescing.

11th January

I think I have been hoist by my own petard. I have been coping with the fact that I have to go into hospital by

ignoring it. It has worked very well. I have been only slightly stressed. Up until today. Today, I have been running about like a lunatic, trying to get a week and a half's worth of housework done in one day. I've been cooking and cleaning, washing and ironing, tidying and arranging stuff all day. I have even managed to put a holiday message on my email, which will reply automatically to people while I am away.

Gosh, I'm clever! It is now 11.30 at night, and I am just thinking about organising my bedroom before I go to sleep. Tomorrow I will pack.

12th January

Claire ill. Got nothing done today. Roll on tomorrow.

13th January

The hospital has rung to say that there is a bed for me, and I am to go in now. I have one bag, a magazine, and my train ticket. Off I go.

***

I slept most of the way up, and have been put into the same ward that I was in last time. The surgeon has been, to remind me what he is going to do (does he think I will have forgotten?), and I have signed the consent form. I am now bored silly, and have time to sit and worry about the operation. The hospital has a huge range of shops and cafes downstairs, so I think I will go and get myself a sticky bun.

I asked about the repeated danger of damage to my vocal chords. He said it was one chance in a hundred before, but the odds had lowered now. I pressed him to be more specific, and he admitted that it was now nearer one chance in ten. Oh well. Too late to back out now.

Post script: went down to Tom's Café and found that they had run out of hot chocolate. How can that be possible? I ate mandarin cheesecake, and bought some crunchy chocolate bars for later.

14th January

It is now late evening. No sign of being tucked in for the night, so I am scribbling a quick note. The blinds are never drawn here, and I can look out at the bright lights of London, across Westminster Bridge, and down The Thames. Why are there so many people still about? What are they all doing? Where are they all going?

The nurse brought me the gown and comedy socks first thing this morning, and suggested I getready, as they sometimes changed the order of the queue. As I was joking about this, and finding my toothbrush, the orderlies came to collect me! I was whisked away, and into the tiny cloakroom they use to 'prep' you. When the anaesthetist had to leave the room, he asked a nurse to sit with me. Whether it was to stop me rifling through the medicine cabinet, or to stop me running away, I don't know.

Anyway, I am back. They are insisting I keep the anti-thrombosis socks on, and I have a drip attached, but there is only one drain (attached centrally), so I am a lot better off than I was last time. This will be the best that I feel for a while, I think, while I am still under the effects of the anaesthetic.

See – I am so used to surgery now, I haven't even mentioned it!

15th January

Feeling sick. The drip has finished, and been removed, but they won't take the canula out of the back of my hand in case they need to use it in an emergency. That's really reassuring. Bad night's sleep last night, due to the amount of light always on, and the moaning of the other patients. Hope that will improve.

The nice doctor came round and explained that everything had gone well yesterday, and that they had removed a thyroid remnant about the size of his little finger, and two more lymph nodes, comprising a lump about the size of half a kiwifruit in total. If I have to get operated on again, my chest will look like I've had a gunshot wound. I quite like that idea. I'll swagger as I walk, and say things like 'Get off your horse and drink your milk'.

Oh, and I fainted this morning. In my efforts to seem cheerful and competent so that they would let me go home, I overdid the speed with which I dressed. So that one backfired on me.

16th January

I didn't get the good night's sleep that I wanted. I woke up crying at one point, thinking that I was turning into a pig.

My feet and face were tingling, like they were turning into trotters and a snout, and my little fingers and ring fingers were stiff and unbendable. Understandably, I cried. A nice nurse came and sat with me. I want to go home!

I am still feeling weepy and fed up with being in here. The tingling on my face and in my fingers (signalling lack of calcium I now realise) got worse as the day went on, despite being given tablets.

The only good thing to happen today was that Colin felt so sorry for me after he phoned, that he jumped on a train and came to visit. Two hours each way. There's a model of true love for you, if ever there was one.

17th January

Hoo-jolly-ray. The blood tests came back OK, and they have let me out, on the proviso that I go and get a repeat blood test done next week. 'Yes, yes', I promise. I was car sick all the way back, and by the end of the journey, we had to keep stopping every ten minutes for me to get out and breath some welcome fresh air. I had an hour's sleep when we got back, and feel a lot better now. I even had some dinner.

18th January

Good day today. I have been taking all the tablets they gave me, and eating all my meals. I haven't exerted myself too much, and been a good girl. The most arduous thing I have done today is to open the huge pile of post which has built up while I was away.

19th January

Well, they say that pride comes before a fall. I don't feel at all well today. My neck is hurting and I feel sick. Early night, I think. I have to ring the consultant and sort out a blood test for later in the week. Why don't I have any servants to do this for me?

20th January

I was very ill last night. By seven o'clock I was vomiting into the toilet. Claire managed to find the number of the on-call doctor, and she came out to see me. I have stopped taking one of the tablets prescribed by the hospital, and she has given me some anti-nausea tablets.

This morning I feel a little better. I am sucking another of the anti-nausea tablets. I will take it easy. I don't know if it's just a reaction to the anaesthetic (after all, I have felt sick after all my operations). Perhaps I'm not allergic to paracetamol after all. It's all too complicated to think about.

Bright point of the day: getting a huge bunch of flowers from work. They are really beautiful. Three cheers for morale-building exercises.

21st January

My neck hurts, and we don't have any more ibuprofen. Shall I take a paracetamol tablet? I think I will just go to bed instead. I have three scars on the front of my neck, where the drain was attached, one entry point, and two stitch marks. I tell Claire it's the drain hole where the drain pipe went in. It gets half a smile.

I took a taxi to the local hospital to have my blood taken,and impressed the nurse with the scars from the summer. If I can't make my fortune any other way, I at least have a budding career as a side-show freak. I was surprised at how little blood she took, being used to the other hospital taking four or five vials at a time. Perhaps they are collecting it in vats somewhere for nefarious practices.

22nd January

I'm getting into the swing of it now. Claire cooked tea today, and I have been trying to hold myself back from doing too much. Yesterday, I did things without realising they would hurt me later on, like watching tv at a slant. I'll just get the hang of it, and I'll be better.

I was reading a psychology book this afternoon, which suggested that feeling nauseous after an operation could be caused by being frightened. We've all heard the expression 'sick with fear', and know about queasy tummies when we are nervous. The author of the book was suggesting that it is not until after an operation that one has time (or allows oneself) to think about what is going on, allowing the reaction to set in. I certainly work my way through the experience by quite effectively blocking it, until I am forced to act. Perhaps next time (will there be a next time?) I should work through my feelings before the operation, and save myself the sickness afterwards. We'll see.

23rd January

All alone today. At least I got a good night's sleep. I have been able to sleep on my side for a few days now, which is a huge bonus, as I hate sleeping on my back. I have been replying to correspondence, and undertaking gentle tidying, like a real lady. I keep looking at my next detective novel, and deciding not to read it. I am only up to watching tv at the moment. I have walked as far as the shop and bought myself a magazine instead.

24th January

Went as far as the post box today. Hurrah for me. Beginning to take enough interest in life to start worrying about all the things I ought to be doing with my time. for a start, I need to write to my GP and get a sick note. I will start a list.

25th January

The superglue they used on my neck has started to peel off, and it looks like a bad case of sunburn. I have picked a bit at the sides, but I am rather afraid that it is going to 'unzip' the scar if I pull it off too early. Eewww.

26th January

The consultant rang today, with the blood test results, and has reduced my calcium tablets from six a day to two a day. Hurrah! That makes me feel as if I am getting better.

27th January

I have been continuing with my programme of relaxation. Whenever I sit down, I take a few moments to breathe deeply. I also now have a huge stock of aromatherapy bath oils and potions from Christmas, which I use regularly. I certainly think that the more expensive ones are worth it. They seem to last longer anyway. I always used to take a book into the bath with me, but I try not to do that now, so that I can concentrate fully and make it a pro-active relaxation therapy session. I like to keep my hands dry, though, and keeping them out of the water would probably be frowned on in true complimentary circles. Ah, well, such is life.

28th January

Had two visitors today – read it and weep! Spent almost all day sitting and chatting, and I am sure it has done me good, because I was beginning to go a bit stir crazy, and want to start doing housework, DIY etc. Got all the gossip from work, and have arranged to have lunch with Bob and Julia at the weekend.

29th January

I decided that I would tackle the ironing pile today. It's not been done since I went into hospital. I thought it would be all right, as my 'injury' is only on the left-hand side my neck, and I am right handed. No such luck. Only five minutes in, and I could feel it beginning to ache. You can imagine how disappointed I was to have to sit down again.

30th January

Got an appointment letter in the post today for my follow-up check. It is during normal clinic times, which is a relief. It means that I am no longer a special case that needs to be seen urgently. Perhaps I am going to get better after all.

31st January

Still feeling very tired. I am finding it hard to sleep at nights, too. I don't know why that is, as I am tired enough during the day. I am also finding that my neck is hurting more. I think that is because I have been doing more than I should, in terms of housework. As locum doctor, I advise less ironing and more television.

February – the month of pancakes and Valentines, in which we say goodbye to our heroine, and wish her well

1st February

I have been peeling more bits of the superglue off my neck. It is gradually coming off on its own, but I am helping it along a bit. It comes off quite easily after a shower or bath, when it is softened.

2nd February

Went out to lunch yesterday. Bad move. I now have a very stiff neck. I think that while I was on my own, I kept my head quite still, and pointing to the front. Being out, I moved it from side to side a lot more, and I am feeling the effects. I had a deep, hot, aromatheraputic, bubbly bath with dimmed lights and candles, to soothe and relax my tired muscles. Not bad, except that I have wet hair where I started to doze off and slip into the water. And so to bed....

3rd February

I am beginning to plan my return to work. I am thinking that I was very tired when I went back in November, and that I should build some half-days into my return schedule. Also, I am feeling guilty about the amount of time I am having off. If I have

to have radiotherapy I will have to have even more time off. So perhaps I should go back as soon as possible now. They are already skimming off parts of my job to other people. I am rather worried that if I stay off much longer, I won't have a job to go back to.

4th February

I saw someone from work while I was swanning around town this lunchtime, and felt obliged to say that I would be back at work soon. I said I would go back 'mornings only', the week after next.

5th February

I got three books out of the library today on 'sudden onset' menopause, for example when brought on by surgery or medication. They say that the symptoms are more acute than those occurring naturally, but also give a long list of remedies to try, ranging from diet and exercise to lists and lists of herbs and supplements. I shall have to try something, as I am still not getting enough sleep, due to hot flashes and insomnia.

6th February

Colin helped me to put up another exhibition today. Once again, I had to stand and watch. Luckily the paper bowls I make are very light, and I can at least carry them quite easily

7th February

I continue to improve. My scar seems almost healed. Perhaps my body is getting so used to it that it has ceased to complain. I have noticed that I am very stiff. I don't know why. I will have to start exercising. Ugh.

Today I realised that Claire has grown from a child into a young woman, and I have missed it. Truly the stuff of romantic tragedies, but heart-wrenchingly painful all the same.

8th February

I read today that people who write, survive cancer better. Something to do with the psychological catharsis of letting it all out, I suppose. So why are there so few books written by cancer sufferers/survivors? Are there boxes and drawers full of unpublished works in lofts throughout the land? Don't people write now that they have television to watch? Or is it just because there's "no call for it"? Who knows?

I realised today that I haven't thought about dying for weeks now. I wonder if it's because I am off work, and less stressed, or because I have got used to the idea now. The reason I realised this was because I WAS thinking about it today. I was hoping I'd last long enough to pay off my mortgage. I have a fifteen year mortgage left, and probably/possibly twenty years to live. I must try to think of a way of altering those odds. It seems unfair that I'll only have five debt-free years.

9th February

I'd like to be known as 'remarkable' when I am gone. As in:' Ah yes, she was a remarkable woman'. What do you think? Better than eccentric. Not so cold as being worthy of respect. So I'd better get on with my life, and do something to earn that title. Time is running out. I think that is why I very rarely sit down and do nothing nowadays. I am very aware that we have limited time on this earth, and need to get as much done as possible while we can. There'll be enough time when we are old and fragile to sit and watch television. Best to be 'up and dong' while we can.

10th February

Having made the decision to go back to work next week, I decided that I should get on with things as I did before. So I have cooked and cleaned, moved furniture, and vacuumed. And boy, does my neck hurt now! That'll teach me. It is late, because I've been slumped in front of the tv drinking two glasses of wine. This means that the hot flushes have started early tonight, and with a vengeance. Just dessserts

More blood taken today.

11th February

They have cut down my lilac tree. The birds still twitter outside my bedroom window of a morning, but not so close. I hear them first thing, sounding the alarm when my cats go past.

12th February

I am getting worried about my appointment on Monday. I think the consultant is going to tell me I have to have some EBR (external beam radiation). I think he is going to tell me I have to have a 'shower' of low-grade beams in a wide arc, to catch an lingering thyroid cells. We'll see.

13th February

A salesman rang today, asking if anyone in our family suffered from arthritis or any similar disease. I told him I had cancer, and smirked at his discomfort. There are upsides to being ill.

14th February

Went out for a Valentine's Day meal today. I wish one could digitally remove skin blemishes, the way you can alter scanner photographs. I did notice that the scare from my neck dissection are almost gone, now, and that my latest scar is almost healed, too.

15th February

Talked to Helen today about how annoying it is to have a problem that is invisible. Having a broken leg gets you loads of sympathy. Having an on-going problem also puts you lower down in the sympathy stakes. People are ready to help and chat in the short term, but patience runs out if the illness lasts more than a week or two.

16th February

Saw the consultant again today. He has adjusted my calcium tablets, as I am still fizzy round the mouth and nose. I now have two each of three different types of tablet to take at three different times of the day. Forever.

I am to have another blood test in two weeks time to test for both thyroglobulin and calcium, one of which is still a bit high, and one of which is still too low.

He is arranging for me to have another CT scan in three months time, when the scars have softened.

And that should be it! No more radioiodine, no external beam radiation, no more surgery, no more constant visits to the hospital 25 miles away. I am grinning from ear to ear, but still not quite taking it in. I know I've been here before, but this time, I am sure it's OK. I will still have to have regular blood tests, and the threat of recurrence never goes away, as it does with many other cancers, but that is something I can live with. The end of an annus horribilus most royal. Not a year I'd like to repeat, and I can't say that it's made me a better person in any way, but it's certainly given me a story to tell.

Roll on old age.

Susan has returned to work full-time, and is currently in remission.

Flying with The Purple Butterfly

Tips on Radioiodine Treatment and the Low Iodine Diet

Contents

Introduction

This section is an attempt to clarify some things about the treatment of thyroid cancer. It is not intended to replace or correct any information given to you by your doctor or consultant. If you are confused or unclear about any aspect of your treatment, these are the people to ask. They are used to patients asking 'stupid' questions, and are more than happy to explain things. They realise that cancer is a very emotive subject, and that information often needs repeating.

The information here is that which I used during my own treatment for thyroid cancer earlier. A lot of it is based on the advice of Ian Adam at Imperial Cancer Research UK. I hope you find it as useful as I did.

I also found the booklet 'Guidelines for the Management of Thyroid Cancer' (by the British Thyroid Association and the Royal College of Physicians) helpful. You can download a copy of the from the BTA website

There are many organisations that can offer help and advice through this difficult time. Some of these are listed in the Links and Organisations section.

Radioiodine Treatment

The main treatment for thyroid cancer is surgery, and most patients will have a total or partial thyroidectomy. This is where the surgeon removes all or part of the thyroid gland.

If you have follicular or papillary cancer, your consultant may advise treatment with radioactive iodine (RAI) after surgery. This treatment should kill off any remaining thyroid tissue in the thyroid area that has been left by the surgeon, and also any cells elsewhere in your body.

Your doctor will explain the procedure in detail to you, and will tell you how the drink or tablet that he gives you will make you radioactive during and after treatment. If he does not have any leaflets about the treatment, you can get them from the British Thyroid Association, or see the Royal Marsden Hospital website. You will need to stay in hospital for about 2-4 days.

Many doctors suggest that you prepare for the treatment by following a low-iodine diet, to make the treatment more effective, and this is discussed in the next chapter. When you come home from the hospital, you will still be radioactive, and should stay away from your family for the times suggested. More information on this can be found in the Yahoo! Support group for thyroid cancer sufferers, in the leaflets mentioned above.

Your doctor will also ask you to stop taking your thyroxine tablets for four weeks before the treatment. This will increase the amount of Thyroid Stimulating Hormone in your blood, and increase the activity of any thyroid cells in your body. This means that when you are given the radioactive iodine, the cells are ready to take it up eagerly.

Some people experience unpleasant side-effects from being off their thyroxine, and from the RAI itself, e.g. constipation, bloating, excessive tiredness, nausea. These can be rather uncomfortable, but should clear quite quickly once you come out of hospital. Tell your consultant as soon as they start, to find out what tricks or tablets will work best to ease your symptoms.

Jobs to do while waiting for your RAI:

- Arrange to have very small children looked after by someone else when you first come out of hospital.
- Agree where your partner is going to sleep when you come home.
- Cook lots of meals and put them in the freezer.
- Sort out books, magazines, puzzle books, jigsaw puzzle, pack of cards, or other games to take into hospital. Check first if they allow you to take them back out again.
- Buy sour sweets to take in to keep your salivary glands working, and pep up tired taste buds.
- Ask if your room has a video/audio cassette player in it, and sort out some favourite videos/audio tapes to take in.
- Buy Patientline cards, or pack a credit/debit card, so you can use the phone. Write out everyone's phone number, with notes of when they will be home.
- Remind people that they won't be allowed to visit you in hospital.

The Low Iodine Diet

Some doctors recommend that patients following a low-iodine diet (LID) for up to two weeks before receiving radioactive iodine treatment. This is to starve the body of iodine, so that remaining thyroid tissue will 'suck up' the radioactive iodine more efficiently. This should increase the effectiveness of the treatment.

There are very few available statistics on the iodine content of various foods, and the information below has been gleaned from a variety of sources. Many of these sources are contradictory, so what you see is a patchwork of information, taking the most stringent recommendations from each source.

It is suggested that you continue to follow the diet for 24-48 hours after receiving radioactive iodine, so that the thyroid tissue takes up the 'poisoned' iodine rather than iodine from any other source. After this, it is saturated, and you can return to your normal diet.

I have included a list of low-iodine foods in a chart that can be photocopied for use in the kitchen, as well as a list of branded ready-prepared foods that can be used. You will probably find many more suitable foods in your local shops, and will get quite used to reading the small print on the labels. You may find that you feel too ill to eat much during this period, anyway.

Invest in a bread-making machine. As well as being a way to avoid commercially made bread without developing arm muscles like a navvy, the bread tastes really good, and is great fun to make.

The biggest problem you will find is being offered food prepared by other people, and having to ask them what is in it. It can make you seem very rude, but when you explain that it is part of your cancer treatment, people are very understanding. It is best to avoid eating out while on this diet.

The basic rules are simple: **no dairy, no fish, and no E127 additive**. Try and stick rigidly to this, and think of the other items as 'extra points'.

Food Allowed on LID Diet

- Small amount of fresh meat per day
- Up to 4 servings grain/cereal/pasta per day
- Basmati or plain rice
- Fresh fruit
- Barley
- Root vegetables, fresh or frozen
- Unsalted nuts
- Sugar, honey, maple syrup
- Black pepper, herbs
- Cola, lemonade, 7Up, Lilt, Lipton Ice
- Herbal tea
- Lemon tea
- Non-instant tea/coffee
- Beer
- Mushrooms
- Whole grain cereals
- Fruit juice
- Cocoa powder
- Matzo or rice cakes
- Homemade bread
- Popcorn
- Sorbet
- Pure sunflower oil, pure corn oil

Food Not Allowed on LID Diet

- Fish/seafood/seaweed
- Milk, butter, cheese, yoghurt, ice cream, whey/buttermilk
- Dried milk, coffee whiteners
- Margarine
- E.g.g yolk
- Sea salt (table salt is OK in the UK)
- Spinach
- Watercress
- Broccoli
- Commercially made bread
- Red dye – E127
- Soy spread/milk/beans/tofu/soy sauce
- Ham, corned beef, bacon
- Crisps
- Canned vegetables
- Spam and salami
- Glace cherries
- Cough medicine
- Liver, kidney,
- Shop-bought bread
- Multivitamins with iodine in
- Chocolate with milk in it, or with soy products added
- Lecithin, Lactose/lactic acid

Branded LID Foods Available in the UK

Note: manufacturers often change the ingredients in their products – please read the labels on all foods before buying/eating them. I found these foods in supermarkets, health food shops, and at www.goodenssdirect.co.uk

PRODUCT	INGREDIENTS
Ecomil Instant Almond Powder Drink 400g	Partially defatted instant almond, corn maltodextrin maltose.
Ecomil Quinoa Drink 1lt	Water, quinoa, agave syrup, corn maltodextrin almond oil.
Ecomil Almond Milk 1lt	Filtered water, almonds, agave syrup, maltodextrin
Ecomil Hazelnut Drink 1lt	Filtered water, hazelnuts, agave syrup, maltodextrin.

PRODUCT	INGREDIENTS
Oatly	Water, oats, rapeseed oil
Evernat Almond Drink	Water, almond, sugar, maltodextrin
Kallo Organic Dark Chocolate Rice Cakes	Dark chocolate coating (cocoa mass, cane sugar, cocoa butter) wholegrain brown rice
Sunsweet Humzingers	Dried fruit, natural flavouring, rice flour
Sunsweet Apricot+	Dried apricot, natural flavouring, sulphur dioxide (E220)
Allinson Just For Bread 5 Seed Mix – bread additive sachet	Chopped toasted pumpkin, linseed, caraway, and poppy seeds, chopped sunflower seed

PRODUCT	INGREDIENTS
Allinson Just for Bread Sun Dried Tomato and Basil – additive sachet	Sun dried tomato granules, sun dried tomato pieces, dried basil
Doves Farm Strong Unbleached White Bread flour	Wheatflour, vitamin C
Puffed Wheat	Wheat
Sugar Puffs	Wheat, brown sugar, glucose syrup, honey, niacin, iron, riboflavin (B2), thiamine (B1)
Jordan's Organic Muesli	Wheat flakes, oat flakes, fruit (raisins, sultanas, toasted wheat flakes, nuts (raw coconut chips, whole roasted hazelnuts) sunflower seeds

PRODUCT	INGREDIENTS
Shredded Wheat	Wheat
Rakusen's Matzo Crackers	Wheatflour, water
Doves Farm speciality flours – Rice flour, Wholemeal, Unbleached, Malthouse, Pasta, Rye, Gluten free, Organic, Wholemeal	Different ingredients in each product. I would recommend the UNBLEACHED strong white bread flour for breadmaking on LID.
Jordan's Natures Wholegrain Almond Nuts Honey Bar	Conservation grade rolled oats, raw cane sugar, honey, rapeseed oil, almonds, hazelnuts, wheatgerm, wheatbran, sesame seeds, sunflower seeds, natural flavourings (vanilla & almond essence)

PRODUCT	INGREDIENTS
Cypressa Popping Corn	Corn
Atora Suet	Beef suet, wheatflour, hydrogenated beef fat
Kallo Organic Thin Sliced Rice Cakes, no added sugar, with sesame	Wholegrain brown rice (95%), sesame (5%)
Orgran No Egg	Potato starch, tapioca flour, vegetable gum (methyl cellulose, calcium carbonate), food acid (citric)
Orgran Gravy Mix	Maize starch, vegetable protein (hydrolysed), onion, vegetable derived monoglycerides

PRODUCT	INGREDIENTS
Ashbourne Organic Ginger Handbaked Biscuits, Lemon	Wheat flour, vegetable oil, sugar, oats, lemon peel, sugar beet syrup, lemon oil, non-organic raising agent (sodium bicarbonate)
Ashbourne Organic Biscuits, Oatmeal & Raisin	Wheat flour, vegetable oil, sugar, oats, oatmeal, raisins, sugar beet syrup, non-organic raising agent (sodium bicarbonate)
Pure with Sunflower Margarine	Sunflower oil, water, palm oil, salt, emulsifiers (sunflower fatty acids), vitamins A, E, D2, B12, carotenes as colour.

PRODUCT	INGREDIENTS
Co-op Double Concentrated Tomato Puree	Tomatoes
Meridian Crunchy Wholenut Peanut Butter – no salt	Roasted peanuts
White Flora – for pastry-making, frying and roasting	Sunflower oil, hydrogenated vegetable oil, vegetable oil, vitamin E

Sample Daily Menus

I am not a nutritionist, and these are menus I put together purely for my own use. I have tried to incorporate general 'healthy eating' rules combined with LID recommendations. The reason I drew up these sheets was so that it would give me one less thing to think about while I was off my medication prior to the RAI. I am not suggesting that anyone follows this list exactly, but it might be a useful starting point if you wanted to write a list of your own, using dishes you normally cook for your family.

Although I have included three weekly menus, this does not mean that you necessarily should follow the diet for three weeks. Two weeks or ten days should be enough.

Week One

	BREAKFAST	MID-MORNING	LUNCH
MON	Fruit juice, porridge, coffee/tea	Biscuit or snack bar, hot/cold drink	Peanut butter sandwich, Vegetable soup, pear
TUES	Fruit juice, toast, coffee/tea	Banana, hot/cold drink	Salsa dip, crudités, hazelnuts, orange, muffin
WED	Fruit juice, cereal, coffee /tea	Apple, biscuit, hot/cold drink	Chicken salad sandwich, vegetable soup, grapes
THUR	Fruit juice, toast, coffee/tea	Muffin, hot/cold drink	Chicken soup, home-made scone/jam, 3 plums
FRI	Orange juice, cereal, coffee/tea	Biscuit or snack bar, hot/cold drink	Hot beef sandwich, salad, apple
SAT	Orange juice, fruit salad, toast, coffee/tea	Banana, hot/cold drink	Chicken Soup and a roll, pear or peach
SUN	Grapefruit, toast, coffee/tea	Snack bar, hot/cold drink	Pasta salad, nectarine

	MID-AFTERNOON	DINNER
MON	Tea/coffee, biscuits	Shepherd's pie, lemon sorbet
TUES	Tea/coffee, biscuits	Chicken stew, new potatoes, baked apple with dates, custard
WED	Tea/coffee, Seeds/nuts	Vegetable curry, basmati rice, banana fritters
THUR	Tea/coffee, biscuits	Roast pork with apple, roast potatoes, green fruit salad
FRI	Tea/coffee, biscuits	Pasta with sauce, porridge topped apples
SAT	Tea/coffee, biscuits	Beef stew with dumplings, melon with raspberries
SUN	Tea/coffee, biscuits	Chicken in the pot, syrup tart

Week Two

	BREAKFAST	MID-MORNING	LUNCH
MON	Orange juice, porridge, coffee/tea	Biscuit or snack bar, hot/cold drink	Peanut Butter sandwich, veg. soup peach
TUES	Grapefruit juice, toast, coffee/tea	Banana, Hot/cold drink, sunflower seeds	Salsa dip, crudités, mixed nuts, orange, muffin
WED	Orange juice, cereal, coffee /tea	Unsalted nuts, apple hot/cold drink	Chicken sandwich, veg. soup grapes
THUR	Grapefruit juice, toast coffee/tea	Muffin, hot/cold drink	Pasta salad, banana
FRI	Orange juice, cereal, coffee/tea	Unsalted nuts, dried fruit, hot drink	Cold chicken salad, Apple
SAT	Orange juice, toast, coffee/tea	Hot/cold drink, biscuits	Chicken soup & roll, scone, peach
SUN	Grapefruit segments, toast, coffee/tea	Biscuit or snack bar, hot/cold drink	Fresh tomato soup, bread roll, banana

	MID-AFTERNOON	DINNER
MON	Tea/coffee, biscuit	Stir-fry beef, rice, Summer fruit sherbet
TUES	Tea/coffee biscuits	Pork chops, potato croquettes, apple snow
WED	Tea/coffee, Biscuit	Vegetable jambalaya, rice pudding
THUR	Tea/coffee, biscuits	Lemony chicken , fried potatoes, fruit salad
FRI	Tea/coffee, biscuits	Vegetable stew, jam tart, custard
SAT	Tea/coffee, biscuits	Turkey curry, basmati rice, banana fritters
SUN	Tea/coffee, biscuits	Roast beef, plum crumble, custard

Week Three

	BREAKFAST	MID-MORNING	LUNCH
MON	Orange juice, porridge, coffee/tea	Biscuit or snack bar, Hot/cold drink	Peanut butter sandwich, pear, veg. soup
TUES	Grapefruit juice, toast, coffee/tea	Banana, hot/cold drink	Salsa dip, crudités, sunflower seeds, orange, muffin
WED	Orange juice, cereal, coffee /tea	Apple, biscuit, hot/cold drink	Chicken salad Sandwich, veg. soup, grapes
THUR	Grapefruit juice, cereal, coffee/tea	Muffin, hot/cold drink	Mushrooms on toast, three plums
FRI	Orange juice, cereal, coffee/tea	Biscuit or snack bar, hot/cold drink	Hot beef sandwich, salad, apple
SAT	Orange juice, toast, coffee/tea	Banana , hot/cold drink	Ratatouille, pear or peach
SUN	Grapefruit segments , toast, coffee/tea	Biscuit or snack bar, hot/cold drink	Pasta salad, nectarine

	MID-AFTERNOON	DINNER
MON	Tea/coffee, biscuits	Irish stew, blackcurrant & apples, custard
TUES	Tea/coffee, biscuits	chicken in a basket, chips, lemon sorbet
WED	Tea/coffee, unsalted nuts	Vegetable kebabs, basmati rice, apricot jelly
THUR	Tea/coffee, biscuits	Pork with plum sauce, roast potatoes, fruit salad
FRI	Tea/coffee, biscuits	Pasta with sauce, melon with sherry
SAT	Tea/coffee, biscuits	Beef beer pot roast, toffee bananas
SUN	Tea/coffee, biscuits	Chicken in red wine, calvados apples, brandy snaps

Recipe Tips

This section does not contain detailed recipes, because I think it is easiest to use the recipes you are used to, and just adjust them to fit the low-iodine diet. This way, you should find that many of your usual foods can be eaten with only slight variation, and that the whole family can still eat together. I think it is important to try and keep as normal as possibly throughout this, for your own sanity, apart from anything else.

What this section does include are tips on preparing some of the meals suggested in the menus above. I went out and bought some coloured stickers before I went on the LID. I then spend an afternoon going through my store cupboard with the list in my hand, and stuck a coloured marker onto all the foods I could eat. If you do this, it makes it is easier when cooking, both for yourself and your family, to see which ingredients you are allowed.

Main Meals and Salads

Shepherd's Pie	Use LID butter and milk in the potato. Don't use a commercial stock cube.
Casseroles and Stews	Use home-made stock, and fresh meat. Check with the butcher that it is not injected with any flavour improvers.
Pasta Salad	No mayonnaise
Chicken Salad	Serve with fresh salsa and chips fried in sunflower oil or skinless new potatoes
French Dressing	Make your own from sunflower oil and vinegar

Light Lunches

Vegetable Soup	There are only a few vegetables on the excluded list. Don't use a commercial stock cube, though. Make your own stock. Add tiny pasta for extra body.
Chicken Soup	Use only fresh chicken from a reputable butcher, and LID vegetables. Make your own chicken stock.
Salsa Dip	Make your own with fresh vegetables. Eat with vegetable sticks, homemade crisps or matzo crackers.
Hot Beef Sandwich	Check the label of the horseradish sauce or mustard if you use it.
Pasta Salad	Pasta tossed with lightly blanched vegetables and French dressing. Don't use mayonnaise.
Mushroom Toast	Use home-made bread and sunflower spread.

Puddings

Rice Pudding	Use almond milk. Try soaking the rice overnight for a really rich taste.
Apple Snow	Omit the egg yolks
Jam Tart	Make your pastry with pure vegetable fat and unbleached flour
Syrup Tart	As above
Lemon Sorbet	Once you have the technique mastered, you can try lots of different fruit sorbets.
Baked Apples with Dates	Substitute any dried fruit for the dates, and add sugar to taste.
Plum Crumble	Use sunflower spread
Banana Fritters	Fry in pure sunflower oil. Use egg white only in the batter.
Scots Porridge Apples	8oz each of sunflower spread and oats mixed with 6oz brown sugar. Layer apple slices on top, pour over 5fl oz water, and bake at 180° for an hour.
Melon with Sherry	Marinade melon cubes in equal quantities of sherry, honey and lemon juice. Serve with roasted almonds.

Calvados Apples	Simmer apples in sugar syrup. Remove apples, and add 3 tablespoons to the syrup while you reduce it. Pour over apples.
Apricot Jelly	Dried apricots soaked and cooked with honey, made firm with the addition of gelatine.

Sweets and Snacks

Peppermint Creams	Don't be tempted to dip them in chocolate
Coconut Ice	No red food colouring – try another colour!
Home-made crisps	Peel potatoes very thinly and deep fry.
Toffee Apples	Use sunflower spread instead of butter.
Popcorn Quick, easy fix of carbohydrate for those missing bread!	Add sugar or table salt – no butter.
Toffee Apples	Use sunflower spread instead of butter.

Biscuits and Cakes

Macaroons	Sugar, almonds, rice flour and egg whites – ideal!
Anzac Biscuits	Use sunflower spread, not butter
Scones	Use unbleached plain flour and sunflower spread. Add raisins but not cheese.
Muffins	Lots of replacements in this one: almond milk, sunflower oil, no egg yolk, unbleached plain flour.
Brandy Snaps	Use LID spread instead of butter. Try them with vanilla essence instead of ginger.
Lardy Cake	Use Flora white fat

Other tips I picked up along the way include:

- Coffee: make real coffee with milk substitute from the list. Add as much sugar as you like.
- Tea: herbal, green or black tea is best, because substitute milk doesn't taste right in ordinary tea. Add lemon, sugar, honey – or all three!
- Cold drinks: 7-Up, lemonade, Sprite, soda water with a twist of lemon, fruit juice, wine/beer
- Cereal: Shredded Wheat, Puffed Wheat, Jordan's Muesli from list
- Toast – use Pure Sunflower spread and marmalade or jam
- Snacks: popcorn with salt, fruit, vegetable sticks
- Biscuits: buy from the list, or make your own
- Porridge: make with milk substitute, and sugar or salt to taste.
- Fruit: interchange the fruit as you like, choosing fresh or dried (if using dried, choose unsulphured)
- Puddings: there are a huge number of sorbets you can made, using fruit, e.g. whites and sugar.
- Bread: make your own bread using unbleached flour. Try not to have too much in one day e.g. don't have toast for breakfast and sandwich for lunch on the same day.

- Egg replacement: use the whites of two eggs to replace one whole e.g., OR 1 tablespoon white sauce, OR half a banana, mashed
- Watch out for 'vegetable oil' as this is often a blend containing soya oil.

Post-RAI Precautions

When you are released from hospital after having your RAI, you will still be radioactive, and you should stay away from other people, especially children and pregnant women. The hospital will give you some guidelines on what you can and can't do. As I understand it, the main hazard to others is from them ingesting radioactivity coming out of you, in the form of sweat, tears, urine, or the tiny drops of spit exhaled when you breathe. If you follow the guidelines on keeping away from people for the prescribed length of time, the other precautions are quite simple – don't let anyone touch you or anything you might have left residues on, e.g. tissues or underwear. And keep washing your hands – it's amazing how often you lick your fingers without realising it.

There are three phases of precaution levels, as the radioactivity works its way through your body. A young person will eliminate the iodine faster than an older person, depending on how well their kidneys are working. As a general rule, multiply the number of gigabequerels (Gbq) of radioiodine by 10 if you are young, by 20 if you are middle-aged, or by 30 if you are elderly. This will give you the number of hours you will be in Phase One. Divide this number by 24 to get the number of days. You will be in Phases Two and Three for 2 days each if you are young, 3.5 days each if you are middle-aged, and 5 days each if you are elderly.

There is no hard and fast rule as to how well your body will work to eliminate the radioactivity for most of Phase One you will be in the hospital anyway. After the first 24-36 hours, you can help your body flush out the radioiodine by drinking lots of water.

Phase One

Sleep alone
Do not cook for anyone else
No kissing
Wash your clothes and sheets separately from the family's
Not more than 1 hour within a metre of other adults
Not more than a few minutes a day within a metre of children under 18
Keep away from pets
Flush paper tissues down the toilet
Try not to lick your fork as you eat, use disposable spoons
Wipe the telephone after use, with a disposable cloth
Keep a selection of pens and pencils for your own use only
No breastfeeding

Phase Two

Only 'dry' kissing
Not more than 2-3 hours within a metre of other adults
Not more than a few minutes a day within a metre of children under 18
No breastfeeding
Keep away from pets

Phase Three

OK to sleep with an adult now
Still be cautious about spitting, dribbling or sneezing on anyone else.
Avoid oral sex

Abbreviations and Definitions

This is a list of some of the terms you may hear during your treatment. Once again, your doctor or consultant is the best person to give you detailed information about any of these words.

Abbreviation	Definition
Anaplastic thyroid cancer	An aggressive form of thyroid cancer
Cancer	Group of cells which multiply abnormally
Carcinoma	Cancer
CT scan	Computer tomography scan which measures tissue density, and so shows up lumps
Dedifferentiatied or Undifferentiated	Cancer which does not respond to radioiodine treatment
Differentiated	Cancer which responds to radioiodine treatment
Follicular thyroid cancer	Less common, usually found in older people

I131	The type of radioactive iodine they use for RAI treatment
LID	Low Iodine Diet, followed before radioiodine treatment, to make it more effective.
Lymph nodes	There are over 200 lymph nodes in your neck. When you have thyroid cancer, it often moves into the lymph nodes. These can be cut out by the surgeon, or treated with RAI.
Metastatic tumours or metastases	A tumour formed when the cancer moves outside the neck to other parts of your body. Thyroid cancer usually goes to the bones or lungs.
Medullary thyroid cancer	A genetic form of the disease
Neoplasm	New cells, sometimes cancerous
Papillary thyroid cancer	The most common kind of thyroid cancer

Parathyroid	Four small glands located behind the thyroid that regulate calcium processing in the body.
PT	Partial thyroidectomy – when the surgeon removes part of your thyroid gland
RAI RAI (cont.)	RadioActive Iodine treatment. Radioactive iodine is introduced into the body either as a liquid, a pill, or an injection. This is taken up by any thyroid tissue in the body, and effectively poisons it. The purpose is to kill any thyroid tissue in the body, which either is already cancerous, or could turn cancerous at a later date
Staging	There are several systems of assessing what stage the cancer has reached. Depending on what stage you are assessed as being, the doctor can give you an idea of how serious your disease is.

Tg Tg (cont.)	Thyroglobulin. The presence of this in your blood shows that there is functioning thyroid tissue in your body. If you have had a TT, there should not be any working thyroid tissue left, so if the Tg levels show in a blood test, it could indicate that there is some thyroid tissue elsewhere in your body. This tissue could be cancerous, and needs to be checked.
Thyca	Abbreviation for 'thyroid cancer'
Thyroid gland	A butterfly-shaped gland in the front of your neck that regulates your body's metabolism
Thyroxine	Hormone produced by the thyroid gland which regulates your metabolism, also known as T4
Triiothyronine	Chemical manufactured by the body from the T4 produced by the thyroid, or taken as a tablet (T3)

TSH	Thyroid Suppressing Hormone. When T4 is taken in large doses in order to keep your Tg levels low, it is known as a TSH.
TT	Total thyroidectomy – an operation to remove all of your thyroid gland.
T3	Also known as triiothyronine. This is the substance your body creates out of the T4 it produces. Sometimes you will be temporarily put onto T3 instead of T4.
T4	A chemical produced by your thyroid gland, also known as thyroxine. If your thyroid gland is removed, you need to take T4 in tablet form each day.
WBS WBS (cont.)	Whole body scan. There are several different sorts of scan, to test whether organs are functioning, or to see where there are tumours or swellings.

Undifferentiated or Dedifferentiatied	Cancer which does not respond to radioiodine treatment

Doses of Radioactive Iodine

In some countries, the amount of radioactive iodine you are given is measured in millicuries (mCi). In Great Britain, we now use Bequerels (Bq) as the unit of measurement. The conversion rates are as follows:

1110MBq is 30mCi = 1.11GBq
3700MBq is 100mCi = 3.7GBq
5550MBq is 150mCi = 5.55GBq
7400MBq is 200mCi – 7.4GBq

Links and Addresses

Internet Links About the Thyroid and Thyroid Cancer:

www.aicr.org.uk/aicrlinks/thyroidcancer
www.baes.org
www.british-thyroid-association.org
www.btf-thyroid.org
www.eurothyroid.com
www.lightoflifefoundation.org
www.papthyca.com
www.thyca.org
www.thyroid.com
www.royalmarsden.org.uk

Internet Support Groups:

'Thyca' and 'Adv-Thyca' on Yahoo Groups – support for thyroid cancer sufferers

Internet Sites About Cancer in General:

www.canceradvice.co.uk
www.cancerbacup.org.uk
www.cancerhelp.org.uk
www.cancerlink.org
www.cancerresearchuk.org
www.clanhouse.org
www.concerningcancer.org
www.macmillan.org.uk

UK Cancer Help Organisations:

British Thyroid Foundation
PO Box 97, Clifford, Wetherby, W Yorks, LS23 6XD
Tel: 0870 7707933

Cancer Aid Listening Line
Ground Floor, Victoria Mill, 10 Lower Vickers Street, Miles Platting Manchester, M40 7LJ
Tel: 0161 205 8446 (office)
Helpline: 0161 205 7780 7.30-10.30 pm

CancerBACUP
3 Bath Place, Rivington Street,London EC2A 3JR
Tel: 020 7696 9003
Freephone helpline: 0800 800 1234

Cancer Black Care
16 Dalston Lane, London, E8 2AZ
Tel: 020 7249 1097

Cancer Research UK
PO Box 123, Lincoln's Inn Fields, London WC2A 3PX
Tel: 020 7009 8820 (customer services)

James MacDonald Cancer Trust
Box 181 Weston Super Mare,BS22 6PJ
Tel: 01934 510230

National Cancer Alliance
PO Box 579, Oxford, OX4 1LB
Tel: 01865 793566

New Approaches to Cancer
PO Box 194, Chertsey, Surrey, KT16 0PZ
Tel: 0800 389 2662

Macmillan Cancer Relief
89 Albert Embankment, London SE1 7UQ
Tel: 0800 808 2020

Marie Curie Cancer Care
89 Albert Embankment, London, SE1 7TP
Tel: 0207 599 7777

NHS Direct Tel: 0845 4647

Tenovus Cancer Information Centre
Velindre NHS Trust, Velindre Hospital,
Whitchurch, Cardiff CF14 2TL
Tel: 0808 808 1010 (freephone helpline)

Printed in the United States
93082LV00005B/49/A

9 781846 851117